CLINICAL CHAPLAINCY

CLINICAL CHAPLAINCY

PRINCIPLES & PRACTICE

DAVID ROTH

VI

This book is intended for education and professional formation. It does not replace clinical judgment, supervision, consultation, or applicable institutional policies and professional standards.

Published by Verbum Icon, LLC

verbumicon.com

First edition, 2026

Paperback ISBN: 979-8-9960247-2-8

CONTENTS

PREFACE: THE RECOVERY OF SOUL

The chaplaincy described in this book is not well-honed kindness, not religious customer service, not a chaplain's private ministry performed under institutional permission, not therapy in clerical dress, and not the ceremonial remnant of an older religious order.

Clinical chaplaincy is the disciplined practice of perceiving persons and human systems differently so that meaning and purpose can emerge in the midst of crisis, distress, loss, grief, or perplexity. It is concerned with meaning, affect, relationship, and system. It asks what for someone is truly—not just supposedly—sacred: what is threatened, defended, lost, desired, grieved, and very likely reorganizing in a life or lives. It asks what is being felt, what is being avoided, what is being enacted, what patterns and relationships are shaping the field, and what sort of help is actually called for.

The chaplain does not provide meaning as though it were a treatment to be administered. Meaning emerges, if it emerges, within a living ecology of person, body, memory, relationship, symbol, culture, and system. The work of clinical chaplaincy is to perceive that ecology with enough depth, humility, and discipline that something previously unseeable, unsayable, or unthinkable may begin to take form.

This book stands in continuity with the public-facing Spiritual Care

Association/HealthCare Chaplaincy Network white paper *Psychodynamic Chaplaincy: Psychological and Spiritual Integration in Healthcare*, for which I was the principal author. That foundational paper helped name a renaissance in psychodynamically informed chaplaincy and spiritual care. This book is not a repetition of that argument. It is a more direct statement of principles and practice for chaplains, supervisors and educators, and institutional leaders who want to know what clinical chaplaincy is, how it thinks, and what it requires. It sets out a path forward for spiritual care as a discipline prepared to meet the demands of our time. It seeks to represent chaplaincy as it could be—and should become—if it is to be a resource of notable value wherever it is deployed.

This is intentionally a thin book. It is not an encyclopedia of psychodynamic theory, neuroscience, anthropology, semiotics, group relations, ritual, religion, or systems thought, though it draws from all of them. It is a field guide to principles and practice. Its purpose is to sharpen perception, supply a durable set of questions, and send the reader back into actual encounters where learning must continue. The book should open trails, not close the terrain.

The book is deliberately aspirational. It describes the most clinically developed edge of chaplaincy, not the average practice of every chaplain and not every legitimate form of spiritual care. It is concerned with the level of work the field should be capable of when suffering is complex, affect is intense, relationships are charged, and institutions themselves are part of the problem. The aim is not to diminish ordinary care. It is to take chaplaincy from where it commonly is toward where it should be.

Clinical chaplaincy is about the recovery of soul. The phrase does not require a metaphysical argument at the doorway. In ordinary religious speech, soul may refer to what endures beyond death, the divine image, the inner person, the seat of conscience, or the object of salvation. Those meanings matter when they matter to the person before us. But for the purposes of clinical chaplaincy, soul will be used more modestly and more concretely—and therefore more universally. Soul is the felt aliveness of a person or system.

Mark Solms puts the clinical point plainly: people suffer mainly from feelings. In the language of this book, soul is therefore not an abstraction added to suffering; it is the felt life in which suffering occurs and from which meaning and purpose may again emerge. Soul is what is at stake when a person says, "I do not know who I am anymore," or when a family argues about a treatment decision that is really about love, guilt, betrayal, and the end of someone's world. It is experienced as consciousness and subjectivity, attached to memory and meaning. It includes the basic affective systems named later as SEEKING, CARE, FEAR, PANIC/GRIEF, RAGE, PLAY, and LUST.

The reader does not need prior knowledge of these systems. Chapter 5 explains only what is needed for clinical attention, and the glossary supplies a compact reference. Their purpose here is not to turn chaplains into neuroscientists. It is to help them notice what feeling is organizing a person or system before reflective language has fully caught up.

The chaplain is not the keeper of soul and is not charged to be the priest or minister of everyone's interior life. A true clinical chaplain is, however, uniquely trained as a participant observer and insightful companion in situations where feeling, meaning, and purpose are being challenged and may become reorganized under pressure.

The book is therefore organized as an ecology rather than a collection of techniques. No person can be understood apart from relationships and contexts; no relationship can be understood apart from the systems and histories that sustain it; no system is without affect; and no affect is without meaning. The chapters separate these dimensions for purposes of attention, then repeatedly bring them back together.

This book begins from several convictions.

First, clinical chaplaincy is broader than healthcare. Chaplains work in hospitals, hospices, prisons, the military, schools, police and fire settings, social organizations, and other places where persons meet systems under stress. Healthcare will provide many of the examples and much of the professional context because that is where much modern chaplaincy has been shaped and where I have principally worked. But the principles belong wherever chaplains work in settings not reducible to congregational ministry.

Second, not every professional chaplain is a clinical chaplain in the sense meant here. Working in a clinical setting does not make the work clinical. Having been trained in a program called clinical pastoral education or clinical pastoral training does not make the work a chaplain does clinical. The principles and practice outlined in this thin volume are intended to clarify how clinical chaplaincy is distinct and uniquely valuable. In healthcare, especially, where chaplains are likely to see fewer jobs and more competition for them, raising the bar on one's own professional abilities and pursuing advanced clinical chaplaincy training may be a wise forward-looking choice.

Third, clinical chaplaincy is not defined by institutional religion. While many no longer identify with named religions, including large numbers who describe themselves as spiritual but not religious, religion has not disappeared. It has moved, fragmented, disguised itself, and reappeared in symbolic systems of body, health, politics, recovery, nation, nature, wellness, identity, sport, fandom, and belonging. The clinical chaplain must learn to recognize religious function rather than merely a religious label or named faith-group affiliation.

Fourth, supportive presence is not enough. Presence may be necessary. It may sometimes be the best a chaplain can offer. But presence can also become a refuge from clinical responsibility. The clinical chaplain must know when and how to listen and observe, when to ask, when to remain silent, when to challenge, when—and more often when not—to pray, when to refer, when to consult, and when to leave.

Fifth, no chaplain should be the sole witness to the meaning of their own work. Case review, peer consultation, and supervision are not merely training exercises on the way to certification. They are part of the ethics of any true clinical practice. Board certification should not become lifelong authorization to do mysterious things behind closed doors without the benefit of others' insight, knowledge, skill, ability, and wisdom.

This book is for chaplains who suspect—rightly so—that the field has become too thin and has not kept up with the times. It is for trainees who need a way to understand why their supervisor keeps asking what is really going on here. It is for board-certified chaplains who know there is more to the work than coverage, referrals, prayers, and patient satisfaction. It is for psychodynamically trained chaplains who want clearer language for what they do and want to round out or deepen their practice. It is for supervisors and educators who want to form clinicians, not merely get folks ready for certification and a job. It is for institutional leaders who want to optimize and better match spiritual care resources to needs.

Clinical chaplaincy is a disciplined practice in helping others in the recovery of soul. It is age-old in its concern for the cure of souls but up to date in its use of contemporary insights from affective neuroscience and neuropsychoanalysis, interpretive anthropology, semiotics, group relations, systems theory, and clinical case learning. It is psychodynamic, intersubjective, and ecological. It works through meaning, affect, relationship, and system. Ever conscious and ever sentient, we do not stop being souls in our various roles as patients, family members, prisoners, soldiers, students, employees, or institutional actors. Whoever we are, wherever we are, we bring our experience of crisis, distress, loss, grief, or perplexity with us. In this sense, all of us could at some time benefit from the care of a clinical chaplain.

The work begins when we stop offering chaplaincy in general and learn to attend to this soul, in this world, under this pressure.

ONE
WHAT MAKES CHAPLAINCY CLINICAL?

The word clinical causes confusion in chaplaincy because it is used in more than one way. Sometimes it means simply that the work takes place in a clinical setting. A chaplain in a hospital is called a clinical chaplain because the setting is clinical. Sometimes it means that a chaplain has completed clinical pastoral education or training. Sometimes it means that a chaplain functions as part of a clinical team. All of these uses have some justification.

But the meaning of clinical chaplaincy in this book is more exacting.

A chaplain, in the broad traditional sense, is a religious or spiritual functionary who works outside the ordinary congregational setting. Chaplains serve in institutions and organizations: hospitals, hospices, prisons, schools, the military, fire and police departments, and other settings where people encounter crisis, distress, loss, grief, or perplexity. The word itself does not guarantee a specific training path, credential, theology, method, or competence. It tells us something about setting and role. It does not yet tell us what quality or kind of care is being offered.

A professional chaplain is usually someone who makes chaplaincy a profession, often with formal training, certification, institutional employment, and accountability to professional standards. But even this term can be slippery. Anyone paid to work as a chaplain may describe the work as professional. Certification bodies may set standards, but standards vary, and the actual formation of chaplains varies even more. Clinical pastoral education or training is not one thing everywhere. People may complete CPE or CPT in programs that differ in depth, method, theory, supervision, expectations, and aims. Some are formed toward deep clinical reflection. Some are trained primarily for coverage, assessment, documentation, and supportive presence. Some are exposed to psychodynamic learning; others are not.

Clinical chaplaincy, as used here, is clinical because of method rather than location. Its method trains the chaplain to perceive differently through disciplined attention to particular persons and systems, learning from cases, formulating what is happening, testing hypotheses, intervening according to role and task, documenting when documentation serves care, and reflecting with peers and supervisors. It attends not only to what people say but to what they enact, avoid, repeat, defend, symbolize, and feel.

A chaplain may work in a hospital and not be clinical in this sense. A military chaplain, prison chaplain, school chaplain, or fire department chaplain may be deeply clinical in this sense. The issue is not geography. The issue is whether the chaplain's practice is disciplined by observation, interpretation, accountability, and care.

Spiritual care names a domain of concern. Clinical chaplaincy names a disciplined way of working in that domain.

This distinction matters. Spiritual care may be offered by nurses, physicians, social workers, family members, clergy, volunteers, friends, and strangers. A nurse who sits quietly with a dying patient may provide spiritual care. A physician who tells the truth compassionately may provide spiritual care. A family member who sings the song a patient loved may provide spiritual care. A rabbi, imam, priest, pastor, elder, monk, or medicine person may provide spiritual care.

Clinical chaplaincy is different not because it is better than all these forms of care, but because it has a particular responsibility. The clinical chaplain must understand the person's meaning-world, the affective currents in the situation, the relationships shaping the encounter, and the system in which the event is unfolding. The chaplain must also understand the limits of the chaplain's own role. The wrong resource, sincerely offered, is still the wrong resource.

The clinical question is not first, "What service can I provide?" It is, "What is really going on here?" Used carefully, that question is a discipline of attention—not a license to interpret people without humility or to find something hidden under every ordinary statement. The first explanation is rarely the whole explanation. What people identify as the problem may be a symptom, displacement, rationalization, or simply the most acceptable version of something harder to say.

The named thing is real, but it is not self-interpreting. A complaint, prayer request, diagnosis, silence, or conflict is part of a larger field. Clinical attention asks what relationships give it meaning, what differences make a difference, and what context would alter our understanding. The map offered by the first description is not yet the territory.

A patient says the problem is pain. Perhaps the problem is pain. But perhaps the pain has become the permitted language for fear. A daughter says the problem is the doctor. Perhaps the doctor has communicated badly. But perhaps the doctor has become the figure onto whom helplessness and anticipatory grief can be directed. A staff member says the problem is the family. Perhaps the family is behaving badly. But perhaps the staff member is naming the only part of the system that can be criticized without touching institutional failure, moral distress, or personal exhaustion.

Clinical chaplaincy does not ignore the named problem. It listens to it as data. Then it asks what the problem may be carrying.

The clinical chaplain is neither amateur therapist nor religious technician. The chaplain's domain includes meaning, affect, relationship, ritual, symbol, moral injury, spiritual distress, religious identity, existential disorientation, family and team systems, and the search for coherence under pressure. This domain overlaps with psychology, social work, ethics, medicine, nursing, community clergy, and organizational life. Overlap does not erase distinction. It requires collaboration.

Clinical chaplains may use psychodynamic concepts. They may learn from the DSM, PDM, neuropsychoanalysis, group relations, anthropology, and pastoral theology. But they do not offer mental health diagnoses unless separately licensed and functioning in that role.

They do not claim every problem as chaplaincy. They do not spiritualize what belongs elsewhere. They do not retreat from what is properly theirs.

The word clinical also implies accountability: a clinical profession does not merely perform good intentions but learns in public enough to be corrected. It has methods, presents cases, receives consultation, recognizes that the clinician's subjectivity belongs to the field, and understands that sincerity is not competence.

Clinical chaplaincy is therefore spiritual care under discipline. It is the practice of attending to persons and systems under pressure in ways that are observant, relational, interpretive, accountable, and appropriately active. It is the work of recovering soul without pretending to own it.

This distinction should be made without contempt. Many professional chaplains who have not been deeply trained psychodynamically still offer faithful, skilled, and humane care. Many clinically trained chaplains also practice poorly. The point is not to create a caste system. The point is to name capability. When language is vague, institutions cannot know what they are hiring, trainees cannot know what they are becoming, and chaplains cannot know what further formation they need.

The field also suffers when the word clinical is used merely as a credentialing ornament. Clinical should mean that the work can be discussed, examined, corrected, and improved. A chaplain who cannot describe the clinical basis for an intervention is not protected by sincerity. A chaplain who cannot say why prayer was offered, why silence was held, why a referral was made, why a note was written, or why a boundary was maintained is not yet practicing clinically in the full sense meant here.

To say this plainly may feel severe. But every profession that serves vulnerable persons must be willing to distinguish role from competence. A badge, title, ordination, endorsement, certification, or job description may authorize entry into the room. It does not by itself constitute clinical practice.

Practice Implications

Chaplain is a broad role, not a sufficient description of competence. Professional chaplaincy and clinical chaplaincy overlap but are not identical. Clinical chaplaincy is defined by method, not setting. The named problem is usually data, not diagnosis. The chaplain must not ask patients to manage the chaplain's task. Clinical chaplaincy requires collaboration, limits, and accountability.

TWO

THE RIGHT RESOURCE MODEL OF SPIRITUAL/PASTORAL CARE

The Right Resource Model of Spiritual/Pastoral Care begins with a simple claim: not every spiritual, religious, emotional, moral, or existential need requires the same response.

This should be obvious. In practice it is often ignored.

Institutions frequently treat chaplaincy as a single resource: a referral is made to 'the chaplain' because a patient is 'spiritual,' a family is 'struggling,' a staff member is 'upset,' a ritual is 'needed,' a death has occurred, or conflict is brewing. The underlying assumption is that chaplains are generalists who should respond to anything that falls under religion, spirituality, meaning, grief, emotion, or distress.

This is convenient for institutions and flattering to chaplains. It is also clinically inadequate.

The Right Resource Model asks: who needs what, from whom, at what depth, under what authority, and toward what end?

It is a collaborative acuity-competency model. Its assessment factors are need, acuity, competency, available resources, and collaboration. The word right does not mean ideal in the abstract. It means fitting for this person, family, staff member, or system at this moment.

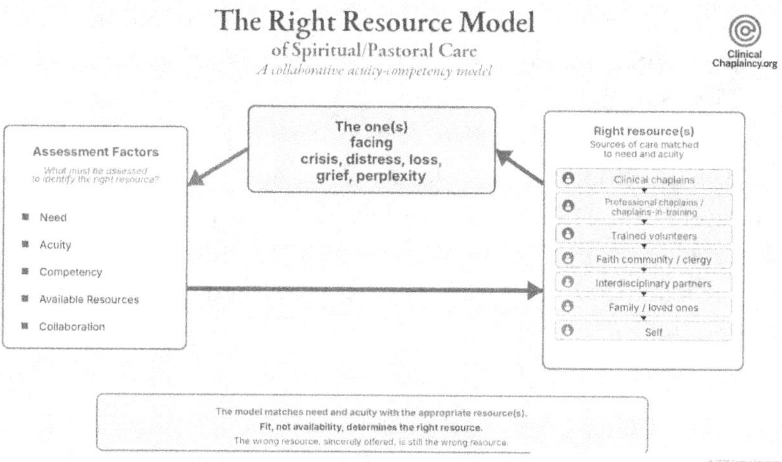

Some situations require ordinary human kindness, information, or the presence of family, friends, elders, sponsors, or community. Others require community clergy, a tradition-specific authority or ritual specialist, a trained spiritual care volunteer, or a professional chaplain. Still others call for a psychodynamically trained clinical chaplain, mental health or ethics consultation, social work, medicine, nursing, security, command, or leadership intervention. Some require no chaplain at all.

The wrong resource, sincerely offered, is still the wrong resource.

This model is not a hierarchy of human worth. It is not a way of ranking patients, families, or staff by importance. It is a way of matching acuity, competence, authority, and task. A volunteer may be exactly the right resource for a patient who wants companionship and has no acute spiritual distress. A community priest may be exactly the right resource for a Catholic patient requesting sacramental care. A staff chaplain may be exactly the right resource for a family that needs orientation, support, and prayer in familiar language. A psychodynamically trained clinical chaplain may be needed when the presenting concern is saturated with unconscious conflict, family system dynamics, traumatic reenactment, moral injury, religious collapse, or institutional anxiety. A therapist may be needed when the issue falls primarily into mental health treatment.

An ethics consultant may be needed when the question is decision-making, capacity, conflict, or moral uncertainty within care.

The model protects patients from chaplain overreach. It also protects chaplains from inflated role fantasies.

BART—Boundary, Authority, Role, and Task—offers a practical way to make the distinctions visible. The following map is descriptive, not a ranking of human worth. It names the ordinary center of each role so that institutions can authorize people honestly and so that referral does not have to feel like failure.

Spiritual Care Volunteer

Task and role. Low-acuity companionship, hospitality, non-clinical listening, practical help, simple supportive practices, and recognition of needs that should be reported or referred.

Authority and boundary. Works by delegated institutional authority and under supervision. Does not independently assess or diagnose, interpret the record, manage complex family or system dynamics, or perform tradition-specific rites without separate authorization.

Community Clergy or Faith-Group Representative

Task and role. Tradition-specific teaching, counsel, prayer, ritual or sacramental care, and continuity with a community of belonging.

Authority and boundary. Authority comes principally from the tradition, community, and the person's request. It does not automatically include clinical training, team integration, access to the record, or institutional authority.

Professional Chaplain

Task and role. Spiritual screening and assessment, empathic listening, emotional and spiritual support, life review, religious accommodation and referral, prayer or ritual within competence, crisis and end-of-life support, staff and family care, team collaboration, and charting.

Authority and boundary. Authority comes from institutional role, policy, credential, and the chaplain's own tradition or endorsement. Professional status does not by itself confer universal ritual authority or competence for high-acuity psychodynamic and system work.

Psychodynamically Trained Clinical Chaplain

Task and role. Provisional formulation of meaning, affect, relationship, and system; work with complex spiritual distress, family and team dynamics, reenactment, moral injury, religious collapse, and institutional anxiety; clinical consultation and case-based learning.

Authority and boundary. Authority depends on institutional role, advanced formation, supervision, and demonstrated competence. It does not make the chaplain a psychotherapist, psychiatrist, ethicist, physician, or universal religious representative.

Role Clarity in Practice

Research helps keep this description from becoming polemic. In the New York Chaplaincy Study, Handzo and colleagues analyzed 30,995 visits and recorded religious and spiritual interventions alongside such general activities as empathic listening, emotional enabling, life review, counseling, crisis intervention, bereavement care, advocacy, and ethical deliberation. Massey and colleagues later organized a chaplaincy taxonomy around intended effects, methods, and interventions. Its intended effects include meaning-making, dignity, peace, connectedness, and care aligned with the person's values. This is substantial work. It also differs from the deeper psychodynamic formulation and system interpretation argued for in this book.

For volunteers especially, BART should be explicit in training. They should know the boundary of the encounter, the authority under which they serve, the role they occupy, and the task they are prepared to perform. Clear limits do not make their care lesser. They make it safer and more useful.

Scope and Limits

The chaplain is not a one-stop all-faiths ministry shop. The chaplain is not a surrogate priest, rabbi, imam, monk, elder, therapist, social worker, ethicist, nurse, or institutional complaint department. The chaplain may collaborate with all these roles. The chaplain may sometimes provide support when the ideal resource is not immediately available. But emergency adaptation is not the same as authority.

Consider ritual. If a self-identified Catholic patient requests communion, a Presbyterian chaplain should not simply provide communion because the chaplain is available and kind. The patient's symbolic world matters. The authority of the ritual matters. The patient's tradition matters. The chaplain can support the request, clarify urgency, contact the appropriate resource, remain present, and help the team understand why the request matters. But the chaplain should not collapse difference in the name of spiritual care.

The same principle applies across traditions. An interfaith chaplain is not authorized to do anything for anyone. Interfaith competence does not mean ritual omnipotence. It means disciplined humility, practical knowledge, reliable referral pathways, and the ability to support a person's symbolic world without pretending to possess it.

The Right Resource Model also helps institutional leaders. Many leaders know they need spiritual care but do not know what kind. They may ask whether chaplains improve patient satisfaction, reduce staff burnout, support resiliency, enhance experience, assist with moral distress, or provide compassionate presence. These are reasonable questions, but they are incomplete. The better question is: what spiritual and pastoral care capabilities does this institution need, for what kinds of acuity, with what staffing, training, and authority?

A small hospice, a trauma center, a prison, a military unit, a children's hospital, a psychiatric facility, a retirement community, a fire department, and a university do not need identical spiritual care systems. They need the right ecology of resources.

The model also changes how referrals are received. When a nurse says, 'The patient wants prayer,' the chaplain does not assume prayer is the task but asks who is making the request, what was actually said, whether the request belongs to the patient, family, or staff anxiety, and what tradition, urgency, and form of prayer are involved. Good care may require prayer, the proper religious authority, a conversation before prayer, or help for staff in tolerating their own helplessness.

When a physician says, 'The family is unrealistic,' the chaplain asks what appears unrealistic—prognosis, miracle, guilt, obligation, cultural expectation, or distrust. The family may need medical clarification rather than chaplaincy, or it may need a clinical chaplain able to recognize that a stated hope for miracle is also a way of keeping love alive. The right resource depends on what is actually happening.

A patient says, "I am not religious." The chaplain does not disappear. Nor does the chaplain force spiritual language. The Right Resource Model asks whether any chaplaincy resource is needed at all, and if so what kind. Perhaps the patient has no interest. Perhaps the patient's symbolic world is organized around military service, music, ecology, baseball, recovery, food, family, work, or bodily discipline. Clinical chaplaincy does not require the person to use religious language before meaning becomes visible.

The Right Resource Model is also a corrective to chaplain anxiety. Chaplains often want to be useful. They may fear that referral means failure. But referral can be the best chaplaincy. Knowing that something is not mine to do is part of clinical competence. The clinical chaplain serves the person and system, not the chaplain's need to complete the work personally.

Assessment begins with need: what is happening, what task is required, and what symbolic or clinical fit matters? Acuity asks how much distress, urgency, risk, complexity, or system pressure is present. Competency asks what formation the response requires. Available resources asks who can actually be reached without confusing availability with fitness. Collaboration asks which resources must work together. Authority remains a governing question throughout: who has standing to act? A person may need comfort from a daughter, sacrament from a priest, protection from a nurse, consultation from ethics, diagnosis from a physician, therapy from a licensed clinician, and clinical chaplaincy from a chaplain trained to understand meaning, affect, relationship, and system.

The model also prevents a common institutional error: confusing availability with fit. The person available may not be the right resource. A chaplain nearby is not automatically the correct responder. A clergy person from the community is not automatically the correct responder. A therapist is not automatically the correct responder. The right resource is not the most spiritual person, the most credentialed person, or the person easiest to page. It is the resource whose competence and authority match the task.

This requires institutions to build relationships before crisis. A hospital should know how to reach local clergy and ritual authorities. A prison should know which community resources are trustworthy and what security boundaries apply. A military setting should know when the chaplain's privileged role is central and when command, mental health, family support, or ethics must be involved. A hospice should know when volunteer companionship is enough and when a clinical chaplain is needed because the family system has become the real patient.

The Right Resource Model is therefore not merely a triage tool. It is a way of designing a spiritual/pastoral care ecology. A strong ecology does not ask one chaplain to be everything. It asks the chaplaincy service to know the field of possible care and to help match need, acuity, competence, and authority.

This is why the model must not be reduced to triage acuity alone. Some low-acuity needs require tradition-specific authority. Some high-acuity needs require no ritual at all. Some urgent spiritual crises are best addressed by a chaplain; others by a priest, imam, rabbi, elder, sponsor, therapist, ethics consultant, or physician. A high-acuity situation may be made worse by the wrong responder. A low-acuity situation may be beautifully met by a volunteer or family member if the system does not overprofessionalize what belongs in ordinary human care.

A mature spiritual care department should be able to map its resources honestly: who can provide companionship, religious accommodation, or tradition-specific ritual; who can assess and diagnose within clinical chaplaincy; who can respond to staff moral distress or consult with leaders; and who can teach, supervise, or say no when a request falls outside scope. Without such mapping, the department may have coverage without capability.

Practice Implications

The Right Resource Model asks who needs what, from whom, at what depth, and toward what end. It assesses need, acuity, competency, available resources, and collaboration while keeping authority and fit in view. It protects against overreach and under-response. It helps institutions build capability rather than merely coverage.

THREE
PRESENCE IS NOT ENOUGH

Presence is necessary. Presence is not enough.

The phrase "ministry of presence" has comforted many chaplains and patients. At its best, it names the gift of being with another person without needing to fix, explain, rescue, or flee. Such presence can be profound. In moments of suffering, abandonment is often the deepest wound. To remain with another without agenda can be holy work.

But presence can also become a copout.

When chaplains do not know what else to say, they may call it presence. When chaplains are afraid to ask a real question, they may call it presence. When chaplains lack clinical formulation, they may call it presence. When chaplains avoid conflict, ritual complexity, staff collaboration, documentation, or referral, they may call it presence. The word can become a pious cover for passivity.

Clinical chaplaincy requires more than being there. It requires disciplined attention, interpretation, restraint, timing, courage, and action. Sometimes the right action is silence. But silence chosen clinically is different from silence caused by helplessness.

Care and love belong to the same clinical field, but neither is useful as sentiment alone. In a December 6, 1906, letter to his protégé Carl Jung, Sigmund Freud famously described psychoanalysis as "a cure through love." For clinical chaplaincy, too, love cannot remain a feeling or aspiration. It must take form as attention, judgment, restraint, timing, and action in response to what this person or system actually needs.

Loving must be operationalized.

Caring and compassion are prerequisites for this work, but they are not yet clinical chaplaincy. The clinical question is what care requires here: whether love asks me to listen or speak, pray or refrain, stay or leave, confront or comfort, refer or remain, document or protect privacy, support the family or challenge its demand, and help the team endure or tell the truth about harm.

Love without clinical discipline can become intrusion. Discipline without love becomes technique.

Working on the margins of vulnerability requires the balance of risk and trust. Every meaningful intervention carries risk. A question may open grief. A reflection may be wrong. A silence may feel abandoning. A prayer may comfort or impose. A challenge may clarify or wound. The chaplain cannot avoid risk altogether. The task is to take appropriate risk in the presence of sufficient trust.

This is especially important in brief encounters, because many chaplain visits are short and the chaplain may have one chance, perhaps two. That reality has led some to conclude that depth has little place in ordinary chaplaincy, but depth does not require lengthy intervention; it requires depth of perception.

In a brief encounter, the chaplain may not interpret transference, explore childhood, unpack theology, or trace family systems. But the chaplain can still notice what is really going on. The intervention may be modest: naming fear, honoring anger, clarifying a ritual need, protecting silence, helping the team understand a symbolic issue, or making the right referral. The depth may be in choosing not to do too much.

Presence is not enough also means that chaplains should stop asking questions that abandon their role. "Is there anything I can do for you?" may be appropriate in ordinary human kindness, but in clinical chaplaincy it often fails. It asks the person under pressure to define the chaplain's task. It implies that the chaplain is available for undefined service. It may produce requests the chaplain cannot or should not meet. It can function as a polite way to end the encounter while appearing helpful.

Better questions arise from clinical attention. "What feels hardest to hold right now?" "What are you afraid will be lost?" "Who understands what this is like for you?" "What do you need the team to know about what this means?" "What helps you remain yourself in this?" "When you say you are at peace, what does peace mean today?" These questions are not scripts. They are examples of questions shaped by chaplaincy's proper domain.

Presence is not enough because prayer is not always care. A chaplain may end with prayer because the chaplain's tradition taught that religious encounters close with prayer. But the patient did not ask. The chaplain feels complete. The patient may feel managed. The chaplain's closure is not the patient's care.

Presence is not enough because good intention does not determine effect. A chaplain may intend respect and still caricature a tradition, intend support and still intrude, intend comfort and still silence grief, or intend advocacy and still overidentify. Clinical accountability matters precisely because intention is not outcome.

Presence is not enough because chaplains work under authority. The chaplain must know role, task, boundary, and competence. A chaplain who acts without authority may harm. A chaplain who refuses appropriate authority may also harm. The question "What is mine to do?" must be joined to "What is required now?"

Presence is not enough because documentation and communication matter. If the chaplain notices significant spiritual distress, family meaning, ritual need, moral conflict, or staff concern, the team may need to know. The chaplain's private meaningful encounter may not be enough if it fails to improve care. Charting should be concise and respectful, but refusing to communicate in the name of spiritual privacy may leave the patient unsupported.

Presence is not enough because the chaplain's work must be reviewed. A chaplain may feel present and helpful while unconsciously avoiding the central issue. Without case consultation, the chaplain may never know. Peer review and supervision are not bureaucratic burdens. They are protections for the work.

None of this diminishes presence. It restores presence to its proper place. Presence is the ground of encounter, not the whole of practice. The chaplain must be able to be with another. But clinical chaplaincy asks what kind of being-with is needed and what must follow from it.

Sometimes the most clinical act is simply to remain. Sometimes it is to leave. Sometimes to pray. Sometimes not. Sometimes to speak a single sentence. Sometimes to call someone else. Sometimes to tell the team that the family is not "difficult" but terrified. Sometimes to acknowledge that no intervention will make this moment less tragic.

Presence becomes clinical when it is disciplined by task, role, authority, boundary, and soul.

In short encounters this matters especially. A chaplain may have one visit, perhaps ten minutes, perhaps less. That does not mean the work is shallow. It means the work must be modest and exact. The chaplain may not resolve anything. The chaplain may notice one thing, ask one question, protect one boundary, arrange one resource, bless one truth, or refuse one false task. Brief does not mean vague.

In healthcare, the course of spiritual care is governed in large part by the course of medical care. The patient may be discharged after a single encounter, transferred before a second, become unable to participate, or return to a community the chaplain will never enter. I have often said that no one has ever been held up from discharge because of ongoing spiritual distress. The line is intentionally blunt. It reminds us that the institution's clock will not wait for the soul's work to feel complete.

Clinical responsibility is therefore not to finish the person's grief, reconcile the family, or restore a world before the transport arrives. It is to identify the next task, intervene in proportion to the time available, communicate what matters, connect the right resource, document what will support continuity, and tolerate unfinished work. The limit of time is not an excuse for vagueness. It is a boundary that makes clarity more important.

Practice Implications

Presence is necessary but not sufficient. Ministry of presence can become a copout when it hides lack of formulation or courage. Loving must be operationalized. Brief encounters can have depth of perception even when intervention is modest. Chaplains should not ask patients to define the chaplain's task. Prayer, silence, documentation, referral, and challenge must all be governed by clinical fit.

FOUR
THE CLINICAL CYCLE

Clinical chaplaincy moves in a cycle: notice, formulate, test, intervene, document, reflect, revise.

The cycle is not mechanical. It is not a checklist imposed on a living encounter. It is a disciplined, self-correcting way of keeping the chaplain from confusing impression with understanding, emotion with truth, good intention with good care, or closure with completion. Like any living system, it remains stable by remaining capable of revision.

Notice

Noticing comes first. The chaplain listens to words, but not only words. The chaplain notices tone, silence, pacing, posture, gesture, contradiction, repetition, avoidance, humor, tears, anger, flatness, timing, who speaks, who does not speak, who watches whom, what objects are present, what religious or cultural symbols appear, what is absent, what the staff has said, what the chart suggests, and what the chaplain feels in the room.

Attend to what is trying to become meaningful—before deciding what it means.

That sentence names the epistemic discipline of the entire cycle. Attention precedes interpretation. The chaplain does not suppress inference; clinical work would be impossible without it. The chaplain delays closure long enough for several possible patterns to remain alive.

The chaplain should be cautious about the feeling that "nothing is happening." Something is always happening. The question is whether the chaplain has learned how to notice it.

Formulate

Formulation comes next. A formulation is not a diagnosis in the medical sense. It is a provisional account of what may be going on. It gathers data into a hypothesis. The patient says he is fine but grips the bedrail when discharge is mentioned. The daughter says she wants everything done but never looks at her father. The veteran jokes whenever grief approaches. The staff says the family is impossible but cannot explain why this family has become the focus of so much irritation. The chaplain asks: what hypothesis best accounts for what I am seeing, hearing, feeling, and not being told?

The presenting problem is not enough. When someone says, "This is the problem," the chaplain receives the statement as important data. But what is named may be symptom, rationalization, displacement, or the only part of the problem that can be spoken without shame. The clinical chaplain does not dismiss the named concern. The chaplain holds it lightly and asks what it may be carrying.

Test

Testing follows formulation. Testing does not mean confronting the person with the chaplain's theory. It means asking a question, making a reflection, or shifting the frame in a way that allows the hypothesis to be confirmed, corrected, or discarded. The chaplain is not trying to win an interpretation. The chaplain is learning whether a perceived pattern has life in the relationship. "It sounds as if the discharge is not just a plan but a kind of threshold." "I notice that when we talk about going home, your hand tightens around the rail." "You have said several times that the doctors are not listening; I wonder what you most need them to understand." "Everyone seems to be arguing about the procedure, but I wonder whether the harder question is what kind of son you want to be right now."

Such statements must be offered modestly. The chaplain is not announcing truth. The chaplain is testing perception in relationship.

Intervene

Intervention means doing what the moment requires within role and authority. The intervention may be silence, a question, the naming of a feeling, arrangement of tradition-specific ritual or community clergy, help to the team in understanding a family's symbolic world, an invitation to speak with an estranged sibling, or a refusal to collude with staff contempt. It may also mean documenting spiritual distress or leaving because the chaplain has become intrusive.

Intervention is not always visible. The best intervention may be restraint.

Document

Documentation should serve care. Charting is not case writing. Charting communicates relevant clinical information to the team. It should be clear, concise, accurate, respectful, and useful. It should not display the chaplain's cleverness. It should not expose intimate material without clinical reason. It should not turn the patient into a theological specimen. It should help the team understand what matters for care.

Charting also establishes the chaplain as a member of the clinical team with something specific to contribute. A useful note usually makes four things visible: the concern, the intervention, the person's response, and the plan. The form may vary by setting, but the logic should remain. "Provided support" tells the team almost nothing. A note that identifies the relevant spiritual concern, what the chaplain did, how the person responded, and what follow-up or resource is needed makes chaplaincy legible without violating privacy.

Case writing is different. A case study is a fuller account prepared for reflection, supervision, peer review, and learning. It includes the chaplain's internal responses, uncertainties, mistakes, fantasies, and questions. Charting belongs to the care record. Case writing belongs to the formation of the clinician. Confusing the two harms both.

Reflect

Reflection means returning to the work with enough distance to learn from it. What did I notice or miss, and where did I rush or avoid? What did I feel and assume; what belonged to the patient, and what belonged to me? How did the institution shape the encounter, and what happened to task, role, authority, and boundary?

Revise

Revision allows reflection to change future practice. Clinical chaplaincy is not improved by experience alone. Experience repeated without reflection becomes habit. Experience submitted to disciplined review becomes learning.

The clinical cycle is especially important because chaplaincy can hide from scrutiny. Much of the work happens behind closed doors, in brief encounters, without witnesses. The chaplain may leave feeling helpful, moved, spiritually satisfied, or misunderstood. None of those feelings proves good work. No one should be the sole witness to the meaning of their own ministry.

This is why case presentation should not end when formal training ends. Professional chaplains, including board-certified chaplains, should continue writing cases for peer review and consultation. Ongoing supervision should be normal, not remedial. The more subtle the work, the more necessary the accountability.

A profession that does not review its cases cannot mature clinically.

The clinical cycle also prevents the chaplain from becoming merely reactive. A call comes: "Patient wants prayer." Notice: who made the request? What exactly was said? Is the patient asking, or did someone assume? Formulate: is prayer desired as religious practice, anxiety management, family expectation, staff discomfort, or chaplain role assignment? Test: ask the patient what would be helpful in their own terms. Intervene: pray if the patient asks and if the chaplain can do so appropriately; arrange someone else if needed; remain present without prayer if that is the better care. Document: note what matters for continuity. Reflect: why did this request affect me as it did? Revise: what will I ask next time before assuming what prayer means?

Clinical work is not less spiritual because it is disciplined. Discipline protects the spiritual from becoming chaplain-centered performance.

The clinical cycle also means that chaplaincy is never simply the encounter itself. The work begins before the visit with referral, chart review, role clarification, and self-awareness. It continues after the visit in documentation, consultation, follow-up, and reflection. A chaplain who treats the visit as the whole of chaplaincy will miss much of the clinical work.

Practice Implications

> The clinical cycle is notice, formulate, test, intervene, document, reflect, revise. The presenting problem is data, not final diagnosis. Charting and case writing serve different purposes. Reflection without revision is incomplete. Case review and supervision are lifelong clinical practices, not merely training requirements. The chaplain's felt sense of closure does not prove that the work was clinically sound.

FIVE
MEANING, AFFECT, CRISIS, AND REORGANIZATION

Crisis as Disorganization

Crisis is not only an event; it is the disorganization of a world.

A diagnosis, death, incarceration, deployment, betrayal, discharge, injury, relapse, institutional failure, or family rupture may change the meaning of everything around it. What had been stable becomes uncertain; assumptions no longer hold; what was sacred may feel absent; and what had been bearable may become unbearable. A person may continue to use familiar words even though the world those words once held together has come apart.

Reorganization may follow, but it is not where crisis begins. Crisis first produces disorder—emotionally, symbolically, relationally, bodily, and often systemically. The person may not yet know what has happened, what can be trusted, or how to act.

Orientation is more than knowing where one is. It is the felt organization that tells us what is real, what matters, what can be expected, how relationships work, and toward what action is possible. When that organization fails, the world becomes strange before a new order has taken form.

Prediction Error and Disorientation

Much of mental life proceeds predictively and outside awareness. We do not first encounter the world as neutral information and then decide what it means. The brain–mind anticipates what is likely through what predictive-processing theory calls priors: expectations drawn from bodily need, memory, relationship, culture, religion, and previous experience.

When experience departs consequentially from what was expected, prediction error—'surprise' in Karl Friston's technical sense—increases uncertainty and may be registered as affective arousal. In Mark Solms' formulation, the quality of the feeling tells us something about a need that has not been met. Crisis is therefore not only an external event but the failure of an established way of predicting and organizing the world.

This is why crisis is felt before it is explained. Breath shortens, muscles brace, the stomach turns, the voice flattens, or the person becomes strangely still. Disorientation is not merely or even principally a cognitive lack of information; it is the emotional and bodily experience of no longer knowing how the world works or where one stands within it.

A crisis of faith, for example, is not necessarily the loss of belief. A person may still believe in God yet no longer know what that belief means after a child dies; a soldier may still believe in duty yet no longer know what duty means after moral injury; a prisoner may believe in forgiveness but be unable to imagine receiving it; and a nurse may believe in care while feeling that care has become impossible. The issue is the disorganization of meaning under affective pressure.

Perplexity deserves its place in the phrase 'crisis, distress, loss, grief, or perplexity.' People may come to chaplains not because they are visibly grieving but because their world no longer makes sense. 'I don't know what to think,' 'This doesn't feel real,' 'I don't know what I believe anymore,' and 'I never imagined this would be my life' all name a world whose organizing assumptions have failed.

Carol Delaney asks students of culture to 'hold on to the disorientation' because it creates mental space in which another world and the relations within it may be perceived. The clinical chaplain may need to occupy that same interval with a person or system: the old cues no longer work, and a new orientation has not yet formed. The task is not to prolong confusion but to resist supplying an orientation so quickly that the person loses the space in which something new might be seen.

Feeling Before Explanation

The work of Jaak Panksepp and Mark Solms is particularly useful here. Panksepp's affective neuroscience identifies the basic mammalian systems that organize experience before reflective thought has explained it, while Solms' neuropsychoanalytic work shows why affect is not decoration added to consciousness but is, in fact, its essence. Feeling is literally at the base of minded life.

Freud had to speculate. Eros and Thanatos were his best attempt to describe the fundamental forces moving humans, but early psychoanalysis had no means of identifying their underlying neural systems. Cross-species affective neuroscience now offers a more differentiated and empirically grounded account in at least seven evolutionarily conserved primary affective-motivational systems, captured in all-caps so as not to limit their meaning to the common, everyday use of the words: SEEKING, CARE, PLAY, LUST, RAGE, FEAR, and PANIC/GRIEF. These inherited subcortical systems generate affect, establish biological value, and organize action; for clinical purposes, they tell us far more about what moves us than Freud's dual-drive theory.

Put bluntly, we do not believe anything on the basis of cortex—'thinking'—first. We feel and are moved spontaneously before we explain. Primary emotional systems establish what is salient, dangerous, desirable, worthy of care, enraging, or grief-laden; the cortex then 'makes sense' of what is already affectively alive by supplying narrative, doctrine, reason, and justification. Belief is therefore never merely a proposition held in the head but a felt organization of reality that reflective thought interprets and elaborates.

SEEKING concerns curiosity, wanting, exploration, and movement toward possibility; FEAR concerns danger, threat, avoidance, and protection; RAGE is fundamentally about frustration and protest when need, expectation, or movement is blocked; and PANIC/GRIEF is based in separation distress, loss, and longing for reunion. CARE involves nurturance, attachment, responsibility, and protection; PLAY involves wrangling and brings joy, flexibility, experiment, and social reciprocity; and LUST concerns desire, in particular erotic and sexual desire.

These systems are not diagnostic labels to impose on persons but maps for attention. They help the chaplain ask not simply what emotion someone reports, but what deep, underlying feeling appears to be organizing this world now.

The seven primary systems are not a complete catalogue of human emotion. Shame, guilt, pride, envy, gratitude, humiliation, moral injury, joy, contentment, and awe, among others, are complex emotions in which primary feeling is joined with learning, memory, relationship, self-reflection, social expectation, and symbolic thought. Shame, for example, is felt but also requires some conception of ourselves as exposed, diminished, or judged—often by an actual or ever-present other—while guilt joins affect with thought about responsibility, harm, obligation, and possible repair.

Earlier experience also remains active through memories and powerful unconscious memory traces. What has happened before may persist as bodily readiness, expectation, affect, image, and relationship even when no explicit memory is available and no hidden story can be recovered. The chaplain's task is not to excavate a secret past or make the unconscious conscious, but to notice when the past appears to organize the present and to work carefully with the form in which it is alive now.

A patient organized by FEAR may not be helped by reassurance until some aspect of safety is addressed, and a family organized by RAGE may experience comfort as dismissal. A staff member in PANIC/GRIEF may present as irritated, numb, or depressed; a caregiver overwhelmed by CARE may collapse under guilt and responsibility; and a person whose SEEKING has been blocked may appear disoriented because no future feels reachable. A system without PLAY may become rigid and unable to imagine alternatives, while LUST, when it cannot be named, may appear indirectly through control, idealization, avoidance, or shame.

Crisis often reveals the difference between the stated problem and the organizing affect. A visitor policy may also become the place where fear of abandonment can speak; a poorly offered prayer may activate religious injury, family loyalty, or an old internal judge; and the demand that someone 'tell the truth' may carry rage at helplessness. The clinical chaplain does not dismiss the stated problem but wonders what else it may be carrying.

Affect also moves through systems. A family may distribute feeling so that one member carries frustration, another faith, another practical competence, and another collapse; a staff team may similarly assign cynicism, tears, procedural urgency, or anger to different members. The chaplain who listens only to individual statements may miss the affective organization of the whole field.

Meaning, Purpose, and Reorganization

Meaning is not a comforting explanation placed on top of suffering. It is the organization by which a world holds together and experience becomes intelligible. Purpose is the forward-directed dimension of meaning: the aims, commitments, relationships, or desired states that organize action and make continued effort feel worthwhile. Meaning helps answer what an experience signifies within our world; purpose asks, given this, toward what can I now move?

Meaning and purpose are not objects the chaplain inserts into crisis. They arise—or fail to arise—through feeling, memory, relationship, symbol, bodily experience, and the systems in which a person is held or abandoned. The chaplain helps create conditions in which reorganization may become more truthful, more livable, and more fully the person's own. In crisis, purpose may contract from a comprehensive life project to the next faithful, loving, necessary, or survivable act.

Reorganization is not always movement toward acceptance, and acceptance can become a cruel demand when imposed too early. Some crises require protest or lament; some require rage to be heard before grief can appear; and some require the collapse of a false meaning before a more truthful one can emerge. Clinical chaplaincy should not rush toward coherence simply because incoherence makes the chaplain feel uncomfortable.

Religious language can conceal affect as easily as it reveals it. ‘God has a plan’ may express faith, resignation, dissociation, family loyalty, or an effort to keep grief from breaking through; ‘She is in a better place’ may be comfort, doctrine, denial, or protection of others from despair; and ‘I cannot forgive myself’ may carry moral awareness, shame, trauma, loyalty to the dead, or punishment sustained by an internal judge. The clinical chaplain listens for the affective current underlying the words without assuming the words are insincere.

The chaplain as an agent of reorganization must therefore be careful. Chaplains do not reorganize other people’s worlds for them; they may name what can be named, hold what cannot yet be solved, protect silence, connect symbols, invite memory, resist false closure, support fitting ritual, or refuse to abandon the person when nothing visible can be done. The task is not to restore a fixed equilibrium but to support a living stability capable of responding to difference, revising expectation, and remaining oneself while becoming otherwise.

Death and dying belong here rather than in a separate compartment, as do deployment, incarceration, miscarriage, dementia, amputation, moral injury, divorce, relapse, institutional betrayal, and the loss of a homeland. Clinical chaplaincy is not a specialty of death but a discipline for attending to persons and systems when meaning, affect, relationship, and system are under pressure. Dying may intensify the work, but it does not create different principles.

This is one reason clinical chaplaincy cannot be reduced to comfort. Comfort offered too soon may ask the person to return to a world that no longer exists and therefore cannot be reclaimed, whereas honest companionship in disorientation may help make feeling tolerable and thinkable until some new meaning, purpose, action, or orientation becomes possible.

The chaplain does not make suffering meaningful. The chaplain helps create conditions in which meaning and purpose may become possible.

Practice Implications

Crisis first disorganizes worlds; reorganization may follow, but it is not where crisis begins. Meaning is not an idea added to suffering; it is the way a world holds together. Primary emotional systems help the chaplain listen beneath stated problems. The named problem may be symptom, displacement, or rationalization. Death and dying are not a separate method; they intensify the same clinical principles. The chaplain supports reorganization without forcing closure.

SIX

THE LIVING HUMAN DOCUMENT—AND ITS LIMITS

Anton Boisen's phrase "living human document" remains one of the most important gifts in the history of chaplaincy. It changed the location of theological inquiry. Instead of treating doctrine, scripture, or ecclesial tradition as the only proper texts for religious reflection, Boisen insisted that persons in crisis are themselves documents to be studied. Human lives, especially lives under pressure, disclose meaning, conflict, faith, despair, hope, guilt, longing, and the reorganization of worlds.

The phrase still has power because it refuses reduction. A patient is not merely a diagnosis. A prisoner is not merely an offense. A soldier is not merely a rank or role. A staff member is not merely a function. A family is not merely a decision-making unit. Each is a living text, written in history, body, relationship, culture, symbol, and feeling.

To read a living human document is not to decode a puzzle from a position of superiority. It is to enter a disciplined encounter with another person's world. The chaplain listens for what gives life coherence, what has been shattered, what is forbidden, what is sacred, what is feared, what is defended, what is remembered, and what is being asked of the soul.

The metaphor of reading is useful, but it has limits. The reading is a map, not the territory. It is made from a particular angle, by a particular reader, at a particular moment in a changing relationship. Clinical rigor does not remove this partiality. It makes the chaplain responsible for it.

Documents can be misread. Texts can be taken out of context. Readers bring assumptions. The same sentence can mean different things in different settings. A silence may signal peace, terror, resistance, exhaustion, dissociation, reverence, or nothing more mysterious than fatigue. A religious phrase may express deep faith, family loyalty, social habit, magical thinking, anger at God, or a wish to end the conversation. The chaplain who reads too quickly becomes dangerous.

Clinical humility begins with the recognition that every reading is partial.

The living human document is not a document written for the chaplain. The person does not exist to provide the chaplain with learning. This is especially important in training contexts where cases are written and presented. Case study is indispensable, but it can become exploitative if the patient becomes raw material for the trainee's development. The clinical chaplain must remember that learning from another's life requires reverence, restraint, and confidentiality.

The living human document also includes the chaplain. The chaplain is not an invisible reader. The chaplain's own life is a text in the room. The chaplain's history affects what stands out, what is missed, what is overinterpreted, and what is avoided. A chaplain who has unresolved anger toward institutional authority may hear every physician as arrogant. A chaplain whose faith tradition centers prayer may experience a patient's refusal of prayer as rejection. A chaplain with unexamined grief may rush toward comfort because grief is too hard to remain with. A chaplain with a need to be useful may ask, "Is there anything I can do?" because doing something protects the chaplain from helplessness.

Thus the living human document requires a second discipline: the chaplain must also be willing to be read. Not by the patient in any intrusive sense, but by supervision, peer review, and self-reflection. What did I bring? What did I need? What did I fear? Where did I become defensive? Where did I mistake my tradition, class, culture, theology, or experience for reality itself?

Boisen's insight was not merely that patients have stories. Everyone knows that. His deeper contribution was methodological: religious experience, mental distress, life history, social context, and meaning-making must be read together clinically. The human document is not divided into spiritual, psychological, social, and medical pages that can be assigned to separate professionals without remainder. The person is a whole, though not a simple whole.

Robert Charles Powell's recovery of Boisen makes this especially clear. The living human document is not an isolated interior. "Co-operative inquiry" reads inner life together with the person's actual social conditions, in all their complexity and elusiveness.

This does not mean the chaplain should address everything. The Right Resource Model still applies. The chaplain may notice a psychological pattern and refer to mental health. The chaplain may notice family system conflict and collaborate with social work. The chaplain may notice medical confusion and ask the physician to clarify. The chaplain may notice religious distress and provide care directly. Reading does not authorize overreach. It guides fit.

The living human document also resists the superficial use of identity categories. A patient may be Catholic, Muslim, Jewish, Buddhist, Hindu, Protestant, atheist, spiritual but not religious (SBNR), or 'nothing in particular.' Such labels matter, sometimes deeply, but none is the document. Everything is local: Catholic in one family does not mean Catholic in another, and Buddhist practice in one patient does not mean Buddhist identity in another. Military service may be the core of one veteran's moral world and a painful residue for another. Race, class, gender, sexuality, nationality, and religion all matter, but they do not relieve the chaplain of reading carefully.

The chaplain reads not to master the person but to serve the person.

Clinical chaplaincy therefore requires an unusual combination of curiosity and restraint. Curiosity without restraint becomes intrusion. Restraint without curiosity becomes polite distance. The chaplain must be interested enough to ask and disciplined enough not to seize.

The living human document is also dynamic. People are not fixed texts. As Heraclitus reminds us, no one steps into the same river twice. Crisis revises persons, and the encounter itself enters the process of revision. Diagnosis, incarceration, deployment, loss, birth, injury, betrayal, forgiveness, and impending death can reorganize a world. What was true yesterday may not be true today. A patient's faith may hold in the morning and collapse by evening. A family may be unified until the decision becomes real. A staff member may appear detached until a particular death breaks through professional armor. Clinical chaplaincy attends to the document as it is being rewritten.

This is why case learning is central. Cases teach the chaplain to read change, not merely content. They teach sequence, timing, relationship, and affective movement. They reveal the chaplain's own participation. They show how a hypothesis emerged, failed, changed, or deepened. They teach that the question "What is really going on here?" is never answered once and for all.

The living human document is not a technique. It is a moral and clinical stance.

The person before us is not an object of ministry. The person is a world. That world can be entered only with permission, humility, discipline, and care.

This is where lean clinical prose matters. The chaplain should not write about another person as though the chaplain has solved them. A case study should keep the person alive on the page. It should show sequence, uncertainty, and the chaplain's participation. The patient or person in care should not become an illustration of the chaplain's favorite theory.

The living human document also includes the social document. Bodies are read differently by institutions. Race, gender, age, disability, class, language, diagnosis, citizenship, incarceration, rank, and role shape how people are seen before they speak. The chaplain must notice not only the person's meaning-world but also the interpretive field into which that person has been placed. A living human document is always read under conditions.

For this reason, clinical humility is not merely personal modesty. It is methodological. It says: I am reading from somewhere. I may be wrong. The person before me is more than my reading. The system is also reading this person, and some of those readings may be harmful.

Practice Implications

The living human document places human lives at the center of clinical theological inquiry. Reading is always partial and risky. Labels do not replace local understanding. The chaplain's own life is part of the clinical field. Case writing must serve formation without exploiting the person. The chaplain reads to serve, not to master.

SEVEN
THE FOURFOLD CLINICAL LENS

The work of clinical chaplaincy can be held in four words: meaning, affect, relationship, and system.

These words do not describe separate compartments. They are lenses within an ecology. Gregory Bateson repeatedly insisted that words and actions have no meaning apart from context and asked, "What is the pattern which connects?" The fourfold lens is this book's practical answer—not a closed architecture that explains everything, but a discipline for resisting the isolation of what only becomes intelligible in relationship.

Meaning, affect, relationship, and system are ways of turning the same living situation slightly and looking again. Each correction changes the others. The aim is not comprehensive mastery. It is perception supple enough to let a more adequate pattern emerge.

These words do not describe separate compartments. They are lenses. In any serious encounter all four are present, though one may be more visible than the others. Meaning asks what world is at stake. Affect asks what is being felt, defended, intensified, displaced, or avoided. Relationship asks what is happening between persons, roles, histories, internal figures, and the chaplain. System asks what larger structures of task, authority, boundary, culture, institution, and community are shaping the field.

The fourfold lens is a way to keep chaplaincy from becoming too small.

If chaplaincy attends only to meaning, it may become intellectual or theological too quickly. The chaplain asks what the person believes, values, fears, hopes, or understands, but misses the feeling that organizes the words. A patient may say, "Everything happens for a reason," but the sentence may be held together by terror. A family may say, "We believe in miracles," but the phrase may be doing relational work: holding guilt at bay, keeping siblings aligned, resisting abandonment, or refusing the authority of a medical team that has not earned trust. Meaning without affect becomes explanation without soul.

If chaplaincy attends only to affect, it may become emotional accompaniment without interpretation. The chaplain notices fear, rage, grief, tenderness, despair, or longing, but fails to ask what world gives these feelings their shape. Fear of death means one thing in a tradition of judgment, another in a family organized around abandonment, another in a military culture of courage, another in a prison setting where vulnerability is dangerous, and another in a secular world where the body is the last certainty. Affect without meaning becomes feeling without world.

If chaplaincy attends only to relationship, it may become interpersonal but not clinical enough. The chaplain notices trust, resistance, attachment, transference, family roles, and the bond formed in the encounter. This matters greatly. But relationship floats unless it is connected to meaning, affect, and system. A patient's warmth toward the chaplain may be gratitude, loneliness, seduction, relief, transference, cultural politeness, or a way to avoid the family. A staff member's irritation may be about the chaplain, or about what the chaplain represents, or about an institutional wound. Relationship without system can become private and naive.

If chaplaincy attends only to system, it may become organizational analysis without care. The chaplain sees task, role, authority, boundary, policy, culture, hierarchy, and institutional anxiety, but may miss the person suffering in front of them. System without soul becomes management. Clinical chaplaincy must read systems without reducing persons to system functions.

The fourfold lens keeps these dimensions together. It shifts the unit of attention from an isolated person or event to a person-in-relationship, a feeling-in-context, a symbol-in-use, and a system-in-motion.

Meaning is not only belief. It includes sacred order, values, identity, memory, obligation, shame, hope, purpose, and the person's sense of what is real. Meaning may be religious or nonreligious, explicit or implicit, stable or collapsing. The chaplain asks: what does this mean to this person, in this world, at this moment? What has changed? What still holds? What is threatened? What cannot be lost without the person becoming someone else?

Affect is not only emotion named in ordinary speech. It includes primary emotional systems, bodily states, mood, intensity, defense, numbness, and the feeling tone of the field. The chaplain asks: what is being felt? What feeling has permission? What feeling is forbidden? What feeling is being carried by someone else? What feeling is being translated into theology, complaint, procedure, silence, or conflict?

Relationship is not only the visible interaction between chaplain and patient. It includes family patterns, staff dynamics, internalized figures, God-images, institutional transferences, and the chaplain's own participation. The chaplain asks: who is present even when absent? Who is being repeated? Who is trusted? Who is feared? What role am I being invited to play? What is happening between us that may tell me something about what happens elsewhere?

Peter Buirski, Pamela Haglund, and Emily Markley aptly call this *making sense together*. Understanding is not extracted from an isolated person by a detached expert. It is co-constructed in a relationship in which both persons affect what can be known.

Relationship also includes what the Soul Group refers to as the ever-present others: persons not physically in the room whose interests, needs, authority, memory, or anticipated responses are active in the encounter. They may be family members, loved ones, clinicians, clergy, supervisors, commanders, community members, the dead, the estranged, or people not yet named. Some are explicit. Others are carried unconsciously as internalized figures or imagined audiences.

Their absence from the room does not make them absent from the field.

System is not only the institution. It includes family systems, religious systems, medical systems, correctional systems, military systems, cultural systems, economic realities, and the immediate organization of the encounter. The chaplain asks: what task governs this situation? Who has authority? What boundaries hold or fail? What roles are assigned? What does the system need the chaplain to do, and is that the right task?

The fourfold lens also protects against common distortions in chaplaincy.

The pious distortion sees meaning but not affect. It hears faith language and assumes faith is functioning well. The therapeutic distortion sees affect and relationship but ignores ritual authority, tradition, and symbolic worlds. The activist distortion sees system and injustice but may underread unconscious conflict and personal history. The institutional distortion sees role and policy but misses soul. The generic spiritual care distortion sees need but not acuity.

Clinical chaplaincy requires all four.

A brief encounter can still use the full lens. The chaplain may have five minutes, not fifty. The chaplain need not perform a comprehensive assessment. But the chaplain's perception can be fourfold. A patient says, "Just pray that I get out of here." Meaning: release, home, control, perhaps rescue. Affect: fear, impatience, rage, or longing. Relationship: the chaplain may be cast as religious helper, magical agent, or safe stranger. System: discharge, medical authority, institutional confinement, family readiness. A simple response may follow: "Getting out matters a great deal right now. Before we pray, what feels hardest about being here today?" Or perhaps, if the patient clearly wants simple prayer in a familiar frame, the chaplain prays. The point is not complexity for its own sake. The point is disciplined fit.

The fourfold lens can also help in case review. If a chaplain presents an encounter by saying, 'The patient was angry,' the group can ask what the anger meant, what affect lay underneath or alongside it, how the patient related to the chaplain, what system pressures shaped the anger, what the chaplain felt, and what task the anger served. The case becomes more than a report; it becomes clinical learning.

The lens can help institutional leaders as well. If a spiritual care department reports only visits, prayers, rituals, and deaths, leaders see activity but not depth. If the department can describe acuity in terms of meaning disruption, affective intensity, relational complexity, and system involvement, leaders can understand why different resources are needed. The fourfold lens turns chaplaincy from a vague service into a clinical capability.

The fourfold lens should not become jargon. The patient does not need to hear it. The nurse may not need the terms. The chaplain needs the discipline. A lens is useful only when it helps us see—and helps us remain ready to see differently.

Clinical chaplaincy begins to mature when chaplains can say not merely that they were present, prayed, listened, or supported, but what they understood: what meaning was at stake, what affect was moving, what relationships were active, what system shaped the encounter, and what care was therefore called for.

Practice Implications

Meaning, affect, relationship, and system form the basic clinical lens of this book. None should be isolated from the others. The fourfold lens protects chaplaincy from becoming merely theological, emotional, interpersonal, or organizational. It can be used silently in brief encounters and explicitly in case review, supervision, and institutional explanation. It gives chaplains a disciplined way to describe what they see and why their interventions fit.

EIGHT
CUES AND CLUES

Clinical chaplaincy depends on the capacity to notice signs.

In Nora Bateson's apt description of her father's method, "The thing was never the thing." The complaint, prayer request, object, gesture, or silence matters. Yet its clinical meaning is not exhausted by what it is called. It becomes meaningful through the relations, contrasts, histories, and patterns in which it participates.

People rarely hand us their deepest truth in a clear declarative sentence. They offer fragments, gestures, repetitions, evasions, metaphors, complaints, jokes, prayers, refusals, silences, and contradictions. Families enact patterns before they can describe them. Staff members reveal institutional anxiety through irritation, urgency, contempt, or helplessness. Patients may speak about pain when fear is the deeper issue, or about God when the question is whether anyone can be trusted.

The clinical chaplain works with cues and clues.

This does not mean the chaplain becomes a detective in the theatrical sense, searching for hidden secrets; it means the chaplain practices disciplined inference. Charles Sanders Peirce's idea of abduction is useful here because it distinguishes among deduction from rule to case, induction from repeated cases to probable rule, and abduction as the formation of a plausible hypothesis from signs that do not yet make full sense. Sherlock Holmes is the popular figure who makes this vivid: small signs, properly noticed, suggest a larger pattern.

Clinical chaplaincy requires abductive reasoning. The chaplain sees enough to wonder, not enough to know. The chaplain forms a hypothesis, tests it gently, and revises it in relationship.

A patient says, "I am fine," while turning away whenever the spouse speaks. A family insists, "We all agree," while one member goes silent. A nurse says, "They are impossible," after a death that resembles another unresolved death on the unit. A prisoner asks for scripture but returns again and again to a particular betrayal. A soldier speaks only of logistics while repeatedly touching a wedding ring. A staff member asks for prayer before a procedure but seems to be asking for permission to be afraid.

None of these signs proves anything by itself. A cue is not a conclusion. A clue is not a diagnosis. But cues and clues invite inquiry.

Attend to what is trying to become meaningful—before deciding what it means.

The chaplain asks: what hypothesis best accounts for what I am seeing, hearing, feeling, and not being told?

Semiotics gives language for this work. Peirce distinguished among icons, indexes, and symbols. An icon signifies through resemblance: a photograph, image, or enactment may look like what it represents. An index points through connection or trace: tears, a tremor, an empty chair, a scar, or a silence may indicate something present by its effect. A symbol signifies through learned convention: a wedding ring, flag, rosary, military coin, scripture, diagnosis, uniform, or ritual phrase carries meanings sustained by a community. Any one sign may function in more than one way.

A tattoo, a worn Bible, a CrossFit shirt, a dietary practice, a silence at the mention of home, or a chair placed slightly apart from the bed may become clinically important. Its meaning is not inherent. Meaning is relational and contextual.

A wink is not a blink. A twitch is not a mock wink. The movement may look similar, but the meaning depends on intention, context, relationship, and culture. Clinical chaplaincy requires learning the difference.

The chaplain must also learn from absence by asking what is not said, who is not present, which words are avoided, what ritual is missing, which family member is never mentioned, and what feeling has no permission to appear. What the patient does not request and what staff do not want to know may also become clinically important. Voids often carry meaning.

Not every absent person is an ever-present other. The question is whether that person's interests, authority, judgment, need, memory, or anticipated response is organizing what happens among those who are present.

When is the best time to rob a jewelry store? When there is a fire next door. Crisis draws every eye toward the obvious emergency. While everyone is looking there, quieter but precious things may be stolen or lost: attention, agency, truth, dignity, moral clarity, and the person's or family's own story. The clinical chaplain attends to the fire without assuming that the fire is the whole case.

This is especially important with religious language. A person who says, "God has a plan," may be expressing trust, resignation, anger, terror, habit, family loyalty, or an attempt to stop further conversation. A person who refuses prayer may be rejecting God, rejecting the chaplain, rejecting performance, preserving privacy, protesting religious injury, or simply not wanting prayer. A person who asks for prayer may want communion with God, emotional holding, a culturally familiar closure, protection, family reassurance, or the chaplain's exit.

The sign is not self-interpreting. Bateson's "difference that makes a difference" is useful here: the clinical question is not merely what differs, but which difference changes the pattern of meaning for this person or system.

Cues and clues also arise in the chaplain's own internal response. The chaplain feels sleepy, irritated, protective, anxious, bored, unusually competent, seduced, shamed, or eager to leave. These feelings may belong mostly to the chaplain. They may also be part of the field. Countertransference is not a problem to eliminate; it is data to be examined.

The chaplain who ignores internal response discards one of the instruments of perception. The chaplain who believes internal response without examination becomes captive to it.

The body is often the first reader.

A chaplain may feel pressure in the chest before recognizing fear in the room. A chaplain may feel pulled to rescue before seeing helplessness. A chaplain may feel anger before noticing that the patient has been subtly humiliating every caregiver. The feeling is not proof. It is a clue.

Abductive chaplaincy must be practiced ethically. A hypothesis should make the chaplain more careful, not more certain. It should lead to better questions, not premature interpretations. It should remain open to correction. The patient, family, staff member, or system must be allowed to teach the chaplain what the signs mean.

Bad chaplaincy often moves too quickly from cue to conclusion. The patient cries; the chaplain assumes grief. The family argues; the chaplain assumes dysfunction. The patient refuses prayer; the chaplain assumes anger at God. The nurse is curt; the chaplain assumes compassion fatigue. The veteran is silent; the chaplain assumes trauma. Any of these may be true. None should be presumed.

Good chaplaincy stays curious.

Cues and clues also help distinguish symptom from source. What is named as the problem may be the part of the problem that has permission to speak. A patient's anger at God may carry anger at a parent. A family's demand for transfer may carry terror of abandonment. A staff conflict over policy may carry grief after repeated losses. A prisoner's theological question may carry shame. A soldier's joke may carry panic. The chaplain does not dig aggressively. The chaplain listens for the deeper organization of meaning and affect.

This is where primary emotions become useful. Is the dominant affect FEAR, RAGE, PANIC/GRIEF, CARE, SEEKING, PLAY, LUST, or some conflict among them? Is the person afraid, grieving, protesting a blocked need, longing for reunion, seeking meaning, trying to care, trying to play, or caught in desire that cannot be named? These are not labels to impose. They are maps for attention.

Cues and clues are not merely about patients. Systems also speak through signs. A unit that repeatedly calls chaplaincy only after conflict has escalated is saying something about its relationship to distress. A prison that uses chaplaincy as a safety valve but not as a source of insight is saying something about authority. A military command that honors chaplains ceremonially but avoids their moral interpretation is saying something about role. An institution that wants spiritual care outcomes but not spiritual care depth is saying something about task.

The clinical chaplain reads persons and systems together.

Practice Implications

Cues and clues are signs that invite inquiry. Abduction forms a plausible hypothesis from incomplete signs. The chaplain must test hypotheses gently and revise them readily. Absence may be as meaningful as presence. The chaplain's internal response is data, not truth. Primary emotions help organize perception. The goal is not interpretation for its own sake but care that fits what is actually happening.

NINE
CLINICAL CHAPLAINCY DIAGNOSIS

Diagnosis is the essential distinctive of clinical care.

This sentence will make some chaplains uneasy. Diagnosis sounds medical, psychiatric, pathologizing, and outside the proper authority of chaplaincy. The concern is appropriate. Clinical chaplains do not make medical diagnoses. They do not diagnose mental disorders as chaplains. They should not turn spiritual distress into amateur psychiatry or use diagnostic language to dominate another person's world.

But if chaplaincy refuses diagnosis altogether, it refuses clinical responsibility.

Diagnosis, in the sense meant here, is disciplined discernment of what kind of problem or suffering is presenting and what kind of response is called for. Pastoral diagnosis, or perhaps more accurately clinical chaplaincy diagnosis, asks what is going on spiritually, religiously, morally, existentially, affectively, relationally, and systemically. It does not replace medical, nursing, psychological, social work, or ethical assessment. It contributes something those fields may not be formed to see in the same way.

In Nora Bateson's film *An Ecology of Mind*, anthropologist Mary Catherine Bateson recalls watching a filmed family-therapy session repeatedly. At first, the child appeared to be making the parents miserable. With further viewing, the mother seemed to be making the child behave that way; then the father, who appeared to be doing nothing, seemed central; then perhaps the therapist. Eventually the pathology could no longer be located in one individual. It was in the pattern of relationship among them. That movement is diagnostic: not the replacement of one culprit with another, but the enlargement of the unit of perception.

Nurses already have a useful basic resource for this part of care. In the fourteenth edition of Lynda Juall Carpenito's *Handbook of Nursing Diagnosis*, the sections on Spiritual Distress and Impaired Religiosity distinguish difficulty integrating meaning and purpose from difficulty relying on beliefs or participating in the rituals of a particular tradition. They identify observable characteristics, contributing factors, goals, and nursing interventions. The distinction is clinically useful. A person may be unable to practice because of hospitalization, privacy, diet, mobility, or lack of an authorized religious leader without experiencing a collapse of meaning. Another person may have full access to ritual while the world those rituals once held together has failed.

Chaplains should know these nursing sections and use their language where it helps interdisciplinary care. But nursing diagnosis is not a substitute for chaplaincy formulation. Nursing screening and assessment may identify a concern, remove a practical barrier, support a practice, or generate a referral. Clinical chaplaincy diagnosis asks how meaning, affect, relationship, symbol, history, and system organize the distress and what response lies within chaplaincy's task. The two practices should meet without being confused.

Powell's recovery of Boisen as a clinician sharpens the distinction. Assessment should be "co-operative inquiry": an exploration of the inner world carried out with the person, not a label applied from outside. The task is understanding toward a reasoned decision about how to proceed.

A chaplain who does not diagnose may still be kind. But kindness without discernment cannot reliably fit care to need.

The first rule is that the named problem is rarely the whole problem. When someone says, "The problem is that my family is not listening," the chaplain listens. But the chaplain also asks what "not listening" means, what feeling is attached to it, what history it repeats, what role the speaker occupies, and what the statement protects. When staff say, "The problem is the patient is noncompliant," the chaplain asks what world the patient is defending, what authority has failed, what fear is being enacted, and what the word noncompliant allows the staff not to feel. When a patient says, "The problem is God is punishing me," the chaplain asks what punishment means in this person's moral world and what guilt, shame, trauma, theology, or family history may be speaking.

The presenting problem is usually presenting on behalf of something else.

This does not mean the presenting problem is false: symptoms are real, rationalizations meaningful, and displacements consequential. The surface belongs to the truth, but clinical chaplaincy also listens for the organization beneath the presentation.

What does clinical chaplaincy diagnose? Several overlapping dimensions.

It diagnoses meaning disruption. What no longer makes sense? What world has collapsed? What sacred order has been violated? What story can no longer hold? What is the person trying to preserve?

It diagnoses affective organization. What primary emotions are active? Fear, rage, panic/grief, care, seeking, play, desire, longing? What feeling is forbidden? What feeling is displaced? What affect is being carried by the chaplain, family, staff, or institution?

It diagnoses relational pattern. Who is being repeated? What roles are fixed? Where is trust possible? Where is authority feared, needed, or attacked? How is the chaplain being positioned?

It diagnoses symbolic and religious function. What symbols carry power? What rituals are needed? What tradition or nontraditional sacred order is operative? What is purity, pollution, salvation, betrayal, forgiveness, judgment, or hope in this world?

It diagnoses system pressure. What task is stated? What task is hidden? What authority is operating? What boundaries are collapsing? What institutional need is shaping the referral?

It diagnoses resource fit. What kind of care is needed now? Is the chaplain the right resource? Is community clergy needed? Is mental health needed? Is ethics needed? Is staff support needed? Is the best intervention a referral, a ritual, a conversation, a note, a silence, or a boundary?

Clinical chaplaincy diagnosis is always provisional. It should be held lightly and tested in relationship. Its purpose is not to pin pathology onto a person. It is to perceive the pattern well enough to determine what care, relationship, boundary, or resource might alter it. The chaplain who diagnoses too confidently becomes intrusive. The chaplain who refuses to diagnose becomes vague.

Clinical Formulation and Charting

A useful clinical chaplaincy formulation should be concise enough to guide action and rich enough to preserve complexity. It should name what has happened or changed, describe how the distress appears to be organized, note the present movement and remaining capacities, and identify the immediate task and appropriate resource. It should also display its own uncertainty. *Appears*, *may*, *seems organized by*, and *at present* are not evasions. They are signs that the chaplain remembers the difference between a hypothesis and a person.

One possible form is:

Following [precipitating event, loss, or change], [person, family, or team] appears to be experiencing [spiritual, moral, religious, or existential disruption]. The world at stake concerns [meaning, sacred order, identity, value, or purpose]. The distress appears organized affectively by [dominant affect or conflict], relationally through [pattern, role, or ever-present others], and systemically by [task, authority, role, boundary, or institutional pressure]. [Symbols, beliefs, practices, community, and remaining capacities] are functioning as [resource, conflict, defense, or site of loss]. The present movement appears to be toward [collapse, rigidity, protest, mourning, repair, or reorientation]. The immediate chaplaincy task is [task], and the best-fitting response or resource is [intervention, restraint, collaboration, or referral]. This formulation should be tested with the person and revised as the field changes.

For example:

Following loss of bodily agency, the patient appears to be experiencing disruption of a moral and religious world in which dependence signifies failure and illness is interpreted as punishment. FEAR is being expressed through anger at staff, while the chaplain is being positioned as an authority who can either confirm or remove the judgment. Hospital routines are intensifying helplessness, although the patient retains strong relational and religious resources. The immediate task is containment, restoration of whatever agency is possible, and clarification of the meaning of punishment—not reassurance or theological correction.

Or:

The family conflict appears organized around guilt and fear of abandonment, with continued treatment functioning symbolically as proof of love. The family's religious hope is genuine, but a goals-of-care conversation that treats "miracle" only as a mistaken prediction may intensify resistance. The immediate chaplaincy task is to help the family speak the love, guilt, and obligation carried by the treatment decision while collaborating with the medical team to preserve clarity.

Or:

The staff request for chaplain support appears to arise less from the patient's stated need than from staff anxiety about the patient's refusal of treatment. The patient's refusal may be preserving agency in a setting experienced as coercive. Chaplain follow-up should clarify the patient's own meaning before offering prayer, persuasion, or reconciliation with the team.

A chart note should communicate what the interdisciplinary team needs: the assessed concern, the chaplaincy formulation, the intervention, the person's response, and the continuity required. It should be concise, clinically relevant, and grounded in the encounter. Diagnosis should not become a pretext for placing unsupported psychodynamic interpretations into the medical record.

Diagnosis also requires negative capability: the capacity to remain with uncertainty. Some situations cannot be formulated quickly. The chaplain may need to say, "I do not yet know." That is better than false clarity. A non-anxious uncertainty can be clinically powerful.

Primary emotional systems give diagnostic depth without forcing the chaplain into psychiatric categories. If the person is organized by FEAR, reassurance may not help unless safety is addressed. If RAGE is dominant, comfort may feel like dismissal. If PANIC/GRIEF is dominant, information may not reach the person until separation distress is held. If CARE is dominant, guilt and responsibility may be central. If SEEKING is blocked, despair may appear. If PLAY is absent, the system may be rigid and unable to imagine alternatives. If LUST or desire is shamed, longing may appear indirectly through control, idealization, or avoidance.

Again, these are not labels to impose. They are diagnostic questions.

Clinical chaplaincy diagnosis should also attend to health rather than treating every strong affect as pathology. Rage may be the soul's protest against violation, grief may be love's truth, fear may be accurate, refusal may be agency, and silence may be wisdom. The chaplain should not diagnose away the person's moral reality.

Nor should the chaplain spiritualize pathology. Some experiences require mental health care, medication evaluation, safety intervention, trauma treatment, addiction treatment, or psychiatric assessment. Clinical chaplaincy diagnosis includes knowing when the chaplain is not enough.

The strongest diagnostic question remains: what is really going on here?

But the question must be joined to another: what kind of care does that call for?

Diagnosis without care becomes analysis. Care without diagnosis becomes sentiment. Clinical chaplaincy requires both.

Practice Implications

> Clinical chaplaincy diagnosis is not medical or psychiatric diagnosis. It is disciplined discernment of meaning, affect, relationship, symbol, system, and resource fit. The named problem is usually not the whole problem. Diagnosis should be provisional, testable, and humble. Primary emotional systems sharpen diagnostic perception. The goal is not to label persons but to fit care to what is actually happening.

TEN
SPIRITUALITY AND RELIGION AFTER RELIGION

Religion is not disappearing. It is moving.

The language of the field has moved with it. Pastoral care is now more often called spiritual care. The newer term reaches beyond Christian, congregational, and clerical assumptions to include patients who are not institutionally religious. That is an important gain. But it can also imply that 'spiritual' names something different from religion: an inward human capacity set against organized belief and institution.

Clifford Geertz's definition dissolves that opposition. It directs the chaplain away from labels and toward the symbolic order by which a life becomes meaningful and real.

Geertz's Definition of Religion — adapted for inclusive language

> "Religion is a system of symbols that establishes powerful, pervasive, and long-lasting moods and motivations in [us] by formulating conceptions of a general order of existence and clothing these conceptions with such an aura of factuality that the moods and motivations seem uniquely realistic."

If you can learn how someone has organized a general order of existence through feeling—what actually motivates them and gives them meaning and purpose—you have a glimpse into their real "religion" or "spirituality." From there, you can see what has been disrupted and begin to help them recover or reorganize what crisis, distress, loss, grief, or perplexity has thrown into disorder.

It is moving out of institutions and into bodies, brands, politics, recovery rooms, gyms, food practices, nation, nature, identity, fandom, therapy, wellness, and private symbolic systems. It is also still present in churches, synagogues, mosques, temples, sanghas, covens, chapels, shrines, homes, and inherited practices. The clinical chaplain must learn to recognize religious function rather than merely religious label.

It is tempting to say simply that religion does not exist. That is too quick, though the provocation is useful. We generalize something as a religion by naming beliefs, ritual practices, sacred texts, authorities, boundaries of inclusion and exclusion, moral obligations, and membership in a community. These abstractions are necessary. They allow us to speak of Catholicism, Islam, Judaism, Hinduism, Buddhism, Protestantism, indigenous traditions, and countless other religious worlds. Without abstraction, we could not teach or think at all.

But abstractions are not the actual life of religion.

Religion is never encountered in general. It is always local. It is embodied in the felt beliefs, practices, loyalties, fears, obligations, memories, injuries, hopes, and symbols of particular persons and communities. A person may identify strongly with a named tradition while living most intensely inside another symbolic world. A patient may say he is a devout Catholic and mean it. Yet his room may be filled with San Francisco 49ers items, and when the priest arrives for last rites during the game, the patient's first response may be, "Hold on, Father, I'll get you at the commercial." This is not evidence that the patient is not Catholic. It is evidence that symbolic worlds overlap, compete, and carry different affective weight in different moments.

The clinical chaplain should not be scandalized by this. Nor should the chaplain reduce it to inconsistency. Human beings are not organized by clean categories. They live in overlapping symbolic systems.

The chaplain can then recognize religious function in unexpected places. Jill Dubisch's work on the health food movement shows how food practices may carry purity and pollution, sacred texts, conversion stories, forbidden substances, temples of instruction, experts, discipline, salvation, and a moralized world of nature against culture. CrossFit may be someone's church. It and other intense body practices such as sweat lodges may provide ritual, community, ordeal, belonging, transformation, testimony, moral discipline, and pastoral-like authority. Recovery communities may offer confession, surrender, sponsor lineage, conversion, testimony, daily practice, and a higher power. Political identity may provide sin, heresy, saints, martyrs, eschatology, and excommunication. Professional identity may function as a moral world. Military service may become a sacred order. Family may function as ultimate concern.

We all have our cosmic nonsense, but for each of us it's our cosmic make-sense.

The sentence is deliberately provocative. It does not give chaplains permission to ridicule what another person holds sacred. It makes the opposite demand. What looks like nonsense from outside a symbolic world may, from within it, establish what is real, trustworthy, obligatory, dangerous, and saving. It may give suffering a place, bind a community, and make a life coherent.

My own Christian inheritance is a useful example. A man condemned and executed as a capital criminal is buried. Three days later, women come to the tomb and find him gone. Later, a man they do not initially recognize meets followers on the road, tells them who he is, remains with them for a time, and then ascends into the sky. From outside this symbolic world, the account may sound like nonsense. Within Christianity it becomes cosmic make-sense: death is not final, defeat may become redemption, and hope can survive apparent catastrophe.

The health food movement, CrossFit, the 49ers, recovery, nation, family, and resurrection differ radically in content. Clinically, the discipline is the same. Meaning and purpose are constructed in symbolic worlds that are felt before they are explained. The chaplain does not begin by deciding whether the world makes sense on the chaplain's terms. The chaplain asks how it makes sense for this person, what primary emotional systems give it force, and what happens when crisis fractures its order.

Robert Charles Powell's study of Queen and Freddie Mercury's dying offers another example. He reads the band's music as a kind of non-ecclesial hymnody for anticipatory and participatory grief: symbolic language for facing death while continuing to live. The point is not that Queen is secretly a religion. It is that music and fandom can perform religious work—organizing feeling, mortality, fellowship, memory, and hope—without presenting themselves as religion.

This does not mean everything is religion in the same way. It means chaplains must notice when something functions religiously.

The rise of 'spiritual but not religious' (SBNR) is one expression of this movement. SBNR does not mean spiritually simple; it often means that a person rejects institutional religious belonging while retaining, recombining, or seeking meaning, transcendence, moral order, healing, ritual, depth, connection, and belonging. The word spiritual is itself a cultural indicator that may signal openness, distrust of doctrine, therapeutic individualism, trauma from religion, longing without institution, aesthetic reverence, body practice, ecological belonging, or simply a refusal to be categorized.

Clinical chaplaincy must neither treat SBNR as a deficit category nor romanticize it. The question remains what is really going on: which symbolic world is active, what carries authority, what is sacred or taboo, what must not be violated, what provides hope, and what gives shame, blessing, or betrayal their force?

The same local discipline applies to people within named traditions. A Muslim patient is not Islam in general. A Jewish family is not Judaism in general. A Catholic nurse is not Catholicism in general. An atheist is not atheism in general. Each person inhabits a local world. The chaplain may need basic literacy in traditions, but basic literacy is not the same as clinical understanding.

This is why the Right Resource Model matters. If a patient has a felt need for a tradition-specific ritual, the right resource may be a person authorized within that tradition. If a patient needs to explore the collapse of a meaning-world, a clinical chaplain may be appropriate. If a patient simply wants someone to share in a familiar prayer, a staff chaplain may be sufficient. If the patient's primary symbolic system is not recognizably religious, the chaplain may still be useful if trained to attend to religious function rather than religious label.

Religion after religion is not less serious than religion before religion. It may be less named, less accountable, and more easily commercialized. It may be more individualistic. It may be shallow. It may also be deeply felt and profoundly organizing. The chaplain who waits only for official religion will miss much of the soul-work of the present age.

This is not a call for chaplains to become experts in every new meaning system. That would simply reproduce the one-stop error in secular form. The chaplain does not need to become a CrossFit theologian, a sports anthropologist, a wellness critic, a political scientist, and a recovery historian before providing care. The chaplain needs enough anthropological humility to recognize that the sacred may be located somewhere other than the expected shelf.

The clinical issue is felt authority: what has the power to bless or condemn, give courage, name purity or contamination, excommunicate, restore order, make suffering bearable, or define the good life? Answers may lead to a denomination, family altar, yoga mat, uniform, sobriety chip, food practice, team logo, flag, or memory of a grandmother's kitchen.

The chaplain should not mock these worlds, and should not romanticize them. Every symbolic system can heal and harm. Every one can hold meaning and become idolatrous. Every one can create belonging and exclusion. The clinical task is not to approve or dismiss the person's ultimate concern. It is to understand the role it plays in the person's life and care.

This way of thinking also helps the chaplain avoid false secularism. A person may say, "I'm not religious," and the chaplain may hear that as the end of their need for or ability to benefit from chaplaincy. But the person may still live by ultimate concerns, sacred loyalties, forbidden betrayals, rituals of belonging, and stories of salvation or damnation. The language may not be theological. The structure may still be religious in function.

Likewise, a person may say, "I am religious," and the chaplain may prematurely assume the content. The label opens inquiry; it does not complete it. The Catholic whose soul is organized by football, the atheist whose moral world is more severe than any catechism, the veteran whose deepest sacred object is the memory of the unit, the wellness devotee whose purity codes govern daily life, and the prisoner whose last remaining dignity is loyalty to a family name all require local reading.

Clinical chaplaincy therefore asks about actual devotion. Not only what do you believe? but what do you serve, protect, fear, repeat, confess, hide, and hope will save you?

Practice Implications

> Religion is never encountered in general; it is always local, that is to say unique to the person. Named traditions matter, but labels are not the living world. People inhabit overlapping symbolic systems. SBNR is not a deficit category. Chaplains must recognize religious function in health, body, recovery, politics, identity, family, nature, work, and other meaning-worlds. The clinical question is what carries ultimate weight for this person or system now.

ELEVEN
AGAINST ONE-STOP CHAPLAINCY

The chaplain cannot be everyone's religious functionary.

This should not need saying. But it does. The modern institution often wants a single spiritual care provider who can respond to all faiths, no faith, every culture, every ritual request, every family conflict, every staff distress, every death, every complaint, and every existential question. Some chaplains accept this role because it feels generous. Some accept it because the institution rewards availability. Some accept it because the alternative is to admit limits.

But the one-stop all-faiths ministry shop is a caricature of chaplaincy.

Interfaith should name a disciplined readiness to work across religious difference, not presumed mastery of many symbolic systems and certainly not authority to perform their rites. An interfaith chaplain should be able to inquire without embarrassment, recognize the limits of partial knowledge, support a person's own practice, collaborate with appropriate community resources, and remain useful when no tradition is named. A shelf of ritual fragments and a superficial vocabulary of world religions do not create interfaith competence. They may only make overconfidence harder to see.

The problem is not pluralism. Pluralism is the condition of the work. The problem is pretending that pluralism can be met by shallow approximation. A little Buddhism, a little Islam, a little Catholicism, a little Indigenous spirituality, a little mindfulness, a little trauma language, a little cultural sensitivity, a little holiday awareness - this can produce the appearance of competence while leaving the chaplain unprepared for real encounter.

Clinical chaplaincy requires something more honest: disciplined approximation.

Competence across cultures and traditions is always partial, but it is not nothing. Chaplains should study traditions, histories, rituals, injuries, authority structures, and local communities; they should know enough not to cause obvious harm, understand why differences matter, and know whom to call. Yet they should remain cautious about claiming cultural competence, which is always approximate and performed in the immediacy of a particular encounter. The real question is whether the chaplain can enter another's world with enough humility, curiosity, and discipline to be useful without caricature.

Beyond cultural sensitivity, but very shy of cultural competence.

This stance is neither ignorance nor relativism. It is clinical humility. The chaplain must learn to ask, listen, ask again, and receive correction. The chaplain must suspend value judgment long enough to work within another's context. This does not mean abandoning moral discernment. It means not mistaking one's own symbolic world for reality itself.

The folly of going native is the opposite error. In anthropology, going native names the loss of critical distance when the observer becomes absorbed into the world being studied. In chaplaincy, it can mean overidentifying with a patient, family, tradition, staff group, or institutional culture. The chaplain begins to speak from inside the other system without authority or clarity. The chaplain may become the family's advocate against the team, the team's agent against the family, the patient's religious interpreter without standing, or the institution's soothing voice while injustice remains unnamed.

Clinical chaplaincy requires proper distance.

Proper distance is not coldness. It is the distance necessary for care. Too far away, the chaplain becomes detached and useless. Too close, the chaplain becomes fused and unreliable. The chaplain must be near enough to feel and far enough to think.

Everything is local. This principle protects the chaplain from stereotype. It also protects the chaplain from abstraction. A Muslim patient may or may not want an imam. A Catholic patient may or may not want communion. An atheist may or may not want a chaplain. A veteran may or may not want to talk about service. A prisoner may or may not understand religion in the way the chaplain expects. A person who says "spiritual" may mean almost anything.

The natural temptation is to generalize. Human beings generalize in order to manage complexity. Chaplains do it too. We cannot function without categories, but categories must remain corrigible. The category should help the chaplain ask better questions, not supply answers.

The chaplain's personal history is always involved. Religious, familial, social, cultural, class, racial, gendered, and professional histories filter what the chaplain notices and how the chaplain interprets it. A chaplain from a sacramental tradition may overvalue ritual. A chaplain from a free-church tradition may overvalue spontaneous prayer. A chaplain shaped by social justice commitments may overread oppression and underread intrapsychic conflict. A chaplain shaped by psychodynamic training may overread unconscious process and underread simple practical need. A chaplain who has suffered institutional harm may identify too quickly with anyone who feels mistreated.

The clinical chaplain does not escape these filters. The clinical chaplain learns to examine them.

One-stop chaplaincy also fails because it confuses respect with substitution. Respecting a tradition is not the same as performing that tradition. Supporting a patient's religious need is not the same as becoming the patient's religious authority. The chaplain can honor a Muslim patient's need for prayer direction without pretending to be an imam. The chaplain can support a Jewish family's need for ritual timing without pretending to be a rabbi. The chaplain can help a Catholic patient receive sacramental care without pretending that all communion is interchangeable. The chaplain can sit with an atheist's moral anguish without smuggling in God.

The chaplain's authority is real but limited. It is the authority to provide clinical chaplaincy within role and competence. It is not universal religious authority.

This has practical consequences. Chaplains should build relationships with community clergy and religious leaders. They should understand institutional policies for ritual accommodation. They should know how to contact appropriate resources quickly. They should document religious needs accurately. They should educate staff about why specific differences matter. They should advocate for patient access without performing what is not theirs to perform.

They should also be honest with patients. "I am not authorized to perform that ritual, but I will do what I can to help arrange someone who is." "I do not want to pretend to know your tradition better than I do. Can you help me understand what matters most right now?" "I can stay with you while we work on reaching the right person." Such honesty is not failure. It is clinical integrity.

Against one-stop chaplaincy is not a call for narrowness. It is a call for precision.

The chaplain should know more, not less. The chaplain should collaborate more, not less. The chaplain should respect difference more, not less. But the chaplain should stop pretending to be a universal spiritual provider. Clinical chaplaincy becomes stronger when it tells the truth about its limits.

Practice Implications

> The chaplain is not a one-stop all-faiths ministry shop. Cultural and religious competence are always approximate. Everything is local. The chaplain should avoid both stereotype and going native. Respect does not authorize ritual substitution. Proper distance allows the chaplain to feel and think. The chaplain's own cultural and religious history must be examined as part of clinical practice.

TWELVE
RITUAL, PRAYER, AND SYMBOLIC ACTION

Ritual is embodied meaning.

It is not decoration added to care after the serious work is finished. Ritual gathers body, word, symbol, memory, authority, and relationship into patterned action so that a difference may become meaningful. It may be formal or improvised, ancient or newly made, religious or not explicitly religious. A prayer, blessing, anointing, silence, song, hand on a shoulder, final salute, poem, or shared breath before a procedure can become ritual when it carries symbolic weight.

Because ritual is powerful, it is also dangerous.

Chaplains often come from traditions in which a religious functionary concludes a gathering with prayer, blessing, or benediction. Because the meeting, service, or visit ends with sacred words, that pattern can enter chaplaincy unconsciously. A chaplain may feel that an encounter is not complete until the chaplain has prayed, in which case prayer may serve the chaplain's need for closure more than the patient's need for care.

Do not pray yourself out of the room.

This is not an argument against prayer, which can be exactly right.

Prayer can hold what speech cannot hold, place fear or grief within a symbolic frame, connect a person with God, ancestors, community, memory, or courage, allow a family to breathe together, mark an ending, bless the body, and give language to what no one can otherwise say.

But the clinical chaplain should always be wary of asking, "Would you like prayer?" The question sounds generous, but it may introduce the chaplain's religious agenda into a moment where the patient has not asked for it. It may also make the patient responsible for accepting or rejecting the chaplain's offer. In some contexts it may be appropriate. But as a default habit it is often more about the chaplain's role-anxiety than the patient's need. It must never be the chaplain's final benediction, exit-the-room strategy.

A firmer stance is needed: do not offer ritual that has not been requested, clinically indicated, or clearly welcomed by the person's own symbolic world. This is not passivity. It is discipline.

When a patient or family explicitly asks for prayer, a ritual need is clear, or the context calls for symbolic action, the chaplain responds. Yet a request for prayer begins rather than ends clinical listening: what kind of prayer is being requested, in whose words and addressed to whom; who should be present; what must or must not be said; and whether prayer is wanted now or after something else has been spoken. The chaplain should not make prayer the default proof that chaplaincy happened.

The same discipline applies to all ritual. Do not offer what is not yours to offer. Do not perform ritual for which you do not have authority. Do not pretend that good intention compensates for lack of standing. Do not collapse another person's tradition into your own available approximation. Do not make "interfaith" mean "I can do anything for anyone."

Authority matters because ritual belongs to a symbolic order. A Catholic patient requesting communion is not merely asking for bread, wine, and kindness. A Jewish patient requesting a particular prayer, a Muslim patient needing support around salat or burial practice, a Buddhist family requesting chanting, an Indigenous patient needing a traditional healer, a veteran needing military honors, or an atheist family requesting no religious language at all: each case requires attention to authority, consent, symbolic fit, and boundary.

The chaplain can help. The chaplain can clarify the need, protect the request from being dismissed, contact the right person, remain present, interpret urgency to staff, and support the person's world. But the chaplain should not claim authority that is not theirs.

This discipline may be called a non-offering stance. It does not mean the chaplain never offers anything. It means the chaplain does not make the chaplain's ritual repertoire the menu. The chaplain attends first to the person's world. If ritual emerges from that world, the chaplain helps determine the right resource. Sometimes the chaplain is that resource. Sometimes not.

The non-offering stance also changes ordinary language. "Is there anything I can do for you?" is usually too broad. It makes the chaplain a general servant of undefined need. Better questions are more clinical: What feels hardest right now? What are you trying to hold together? What gives you strength? Are there practices, people, or prayers from your own life that would be important now? Is there someone from your tradition or community you would want us to contact? What would feel respectful here?

These questions do not force ritual. They make room for it.

Ritual can also be secular or hybrid. A firefighter's bell, a military salute, a song from home, a family recipe, a sobriety coin, or a child's drawing may carry sacred weight. The chaplain should not dismiss such symbols because they are not traditionally religious. Nor should the chaplain manipulate them as though any symbol can be used freely. The question remains: whose symbol is this, what does it carry, and what authority do I have in relation to it?

Ritual should not be used to close prematurely. Families sometimes ask for prayer when what is needed first is truth. Staff may request ritual because they cannot bear helplessness. Patients may ask for blessing while also needing to speak anger. The chaplain should not refuse ritual cynically, but neither should the chaplain allow ritual to cover what still needs attention.

Good ritual does not erase reality. It helps people stand in relation to reality.

Clinical chaplaincy therefore treats ritual as symbolic action under discipline. Prayer, blessing, silence, sacrament, lament, touch, farewell, and improvised acts are not chaplaincy ornaments. They are serious interventions. Serious interventions require consent, authority, timing, humility, and fit.

The non-offering stance may feel like withholding care to chaplains formed to offer prayer. But restraint protects the other person's symbolic world. The chaplain is silent not from emptiness, but to discover what may actually be needed.

There are times when the chaplain may appropriately initiate a ritual possibility. A family may be so overwhelmed that it cannot ask. A patient may not know that a resource is available. A staff team may need a communal pause after repeated deaths. Even then, the offer should be specific, modest, and grounded in what has been heard: "Some families find it helpful to have a prayer from their own tradition or a moment of silence. Would anything like that fit for you?" This is different from the habitual closing question, "Would you like me to pray?"

The difference is not merely wording. It is stance. One centers the chaplain's act. The other centers the person's world and leaves room for refusal, redirection, or a different resource.

Symbolic action also has timing. A blessing before truth may become evasion. A prayer before anger may silence protest. A ritual before consent may become intrusion. A silence held too long may become abandonment. The clinical chaplain must feel the moment without assuming that every intense moment is a ritual moment.

The chaplain must also understand that refusal of prayer may be sacred. Some patients refuse because they are angry at God. Some refuse because they do not share the chaplain's tradition. Some refuse because religious language has been used to harm them. Some refuse because silence is more truthful. Some refuse because they do not want to manage the chaplain. A refusal should not be treated as failure. It is information and possibly care.

Nor should consent be assumed from politeness. Patients often say yes to chaplains because they are vulnerable, dependent, courteous, frightened, or unsure what refusal would mean. A patient who says yes may still be accommodating the chaplain. This is why routine offering is ethically complicated. Power in chaplaincy is often soft, but it is still power.

Ritual authority is not only formal. A grandmother may have authority to sing a song that no chaplain could sing. A unit commander may have authority to speak words a chaplain should not speak. A prison elder may have authority in a pod that no staff member recognizes. A sponsor may have authority for a person in recovery. The clinical chaplain respects formal religious authority, but also listens for lived symbolic authority.

Practice Implications

> Prayer is not the chaplain's proof of usefulness. The chaplain should not pray themselves out of the room. Ritual requires consent, authority, timing, and symbolic fit. Interfaith competence is not ritual omnipotence. The non-offering stance protects the patient's world from the chaplain's need to act. Good ritual helps people stand in relation to reality rather than escape it.

THIRTEEN
THE CHAPLAIN IN THE FIELD

The chaplain is always part of the clinical field.

Every encounter is radically local. This person has not been met before in precisely this configuration of body, memory, relationship, time, institution, and pressure; even a familiar person is not the same person in the same river. Clinical experience matters, but it must never become permission to substitute a previous case for the one now occurring.

This is both obvious and often denied. Chaplains enter rooms as bodies, histories, voices, authorities, symbols, genders, races, ages, classes, religious representatives, institutional agents, strangers, helpers, threats, comforts, and projections. The patient does not meet an abstract spiritual care provider. The patient meets this chaplain.

The chaplain also meets the patient through personal history. Clinical chaplaincy requires a known, questioned, and supervised self.

The self is the principal instrument of clinical chaplaincy. Instruments require tuning.

A chaplain's history filters perception because we do not observe from outside the ecology; our observing enters it. Family roles shape what feels normal, religious formation what feels sacred or offensive, class location assumptions about authority and speech, and gender and sexuality experiences of safety, attraction, fear, and projection. Race and culture shape what is noticed or missed, while personal grief and shame shape our responses to grief and shame. The chaplain's body carries its own archive.

This does not disqualify the chaplain. It makes reflection necessary.

Transference and countertransference are not exotic psychoanalytic luxuries. They are everyday clinical realities. Patients and families respond to the chaplain through prior relationships, fantasies, hopes, injuries, and cultural expectations. The chaplain may become mother, father, priest, judge, betrayer, rescuer, bureaucrat, God-representative, outsider, insider, or witness. The chaplain responds through the chaplain's own patterns. The patient who demands may evoke the chaplain's compliance or defiance. The grieving spouse may evoke rescue. The angry family may evoke fear. The seductive patient may evoke shame, excitement, avoidance, or moralism.

None of this means the encounter is unreal. It means the encounter has depth.

Projection is especially common in chaplaincy because the role is symbolically loaded. People have expectations about chaplains as a group. Some expect prayer, judgment, comfort, irrelevance, moral authority, institutional loyalty, religious intrusion, kindness, hypocrisy, or magic. The chaplain may also have fantasies about what others expect. A chaplain may imagine a patient wants prayer because the chaplain needs to be wanted as a religious figure. A chaplain may imagine staff disdain because the chaplain feels professionally insecure. A chaplain may imagine being indispensable because the chaplain fears being marginal.

Clinical practice requires examining both projections others may have about us and our imaginings about them.

Projective identification names a more relational process. A feeling or role is not merely attributed to another person; the interaction exerts pressure on that person to carry it, feel it, or perform it. A family that experiences authority as abandoning may repeatedly position the chaplain as another rejecting authority until the chaplain begins to feel cold or eager to escape. A team unable to bear helplessness may place it in the chaplain, who then feels compelled to rescue the family or supply spiritual closure. The chaplain's response is not proof that this is what has happened. It is data to be tested, preferably in supervision, before it becomes action.

The inner judge should not be underestimated. Chaplains often meet persons in the territory of guilt, obligation, punishment, worthiness, judgment, and moral failure. But the chaplain must remember: my inner judge is not yours, and it is definitely not theirs. A chaplain's internal moral authority may be severe or permissive, religious or secular, perfectionistic or rebellious. Patients and families have their own internal judges. Institutions have them too, expressed through policy, quality metrics, professional norms, risk management, and moral narratives about care.

Clinical chaplaincy asks how guilt, shame, duty, and moral authority are operating in the field.

Erotic transference must be named without shame. Chaplains work in intimate settings. Vulnerability, dependence, gratitude, admiration, fear, touch, prayer, secrecy, and emotional exposure can produce erotic currents. These may be subtle or explicit. They may arise in patients, family members, staff, or chaplains. Denial makes them more dangerous. Moral panic also makes them more dangerous. Honesty without shame is the safer path.

The clinical chaplain notices attraction, longing, rescuing fantasies, specialness, and boundary pressure. The chaplain brings them to supervision or consultation. The chaplain does not act them out. The chaplain does not hide behind piety. The chaplain does not imagine that ordination, certification, age, or good intention removes erotic complexity from human encounter.

Chaplaincy without memory or desire is a useful stance if properly understood. It does not mean the chaplain has no memory, no desire, no history, and no hope. That would be impossible. It means the chaplain enters without needing the person to become the chaplain's theory, ministry success, theological vindication, emotional rescue, or proof of competence. Bring your whole self, your whole self; do not bring your agenda.

Memory and desire distort when unexamined. The chaplain remembers a similar patient and assumes similarity. The chaplain desires a good outcome and presses toward it. The chaplain wants reconciliation, prayer, peace, insight, gratitude, or tears. The chaplain wants the family to stop fighting, the patient to accept dying, the staff to value chaplaincy, the institution to recognize depth. These desires may be understandable. They may also interfere with care.

The meta-stance is reflexivity: including self as object. The chaplain observes the encounter while also examining personal participation by asking what role is being taken, what is being felt or avoided, what outcome is desired or feared, and how the chaplain may be shaping the field being studied.

This self-observation should not become narcissistic. The patient is not a mirror for the chaplain's self-analysis. But without reflexivity, the chaplain becomes an unexamined force in vulnerable spaces.

Clinical chaplains also need boundaries. Boundaries are not merely rules against misconduct. They make care possible. Time, touch, disclosure, role, availability, confidentiality, documentation, and follow-up all require boundaries. A boundary may be too rigid or too porous. The chaplain who never self-discloses may hide behind role. The chaplain who self-discloses too much may burden the patient. The chaplain who is always available may be meeting the chaplain's need to be needed. The chaplain who is rarely available may be avoiding intimacy.

Boundaries are clinical instruments.

The chaplain's authority must also be examined. Chaplains often feel marginal in institutions. This can produce either timidity or overcompensation. A chaplain may avoid speaking clinically because physicians are present. Another may claim spiritual authority too broadly because the role feels insecure. The clinical chaplain must take up appropriate authority: neither abdicated nor inflated.

The use of self is not self-expression. It is disciplined availability.

The patient does not need the chaplain's unprocessed material. The patient needs the chaplain's formed self: responsive, reflective, grounded, curious, boundaried, and accountable. Formation is the slow work by which the chaplain becomes a more reliable instrument.

The clinical field is therefore not only "out there." It includes the chaplain's body, memory, theology, class, culture, losses, loves, judgments, fatigue, and hope. The better trained chaplain is not the one without such material. The better trained chaplain is the one who can notice it early enough that it does not secretly run the care.

Practice Implications

> The chaplain is always part of the clinical field. Use of self requires self-knowledge, supervision, and accountability. Transference, countertransference, projection, inner judgment, shame, attraction, and boundary pressure are ordinary clinical realities. Chaplaincy without memory or desire means bringing the whole self without bringing an agenda. Boundaries and authority are instruments of care.

FOURTEEN
TRAB-S

Clinical chaplaincy happens in systems.

A patient room is a system. A family is a system. A unit is a system. A prison tier, military command, hospice team, trauma bay, school, congregation, board, and nonprofit are systems. The chaplain is never simply with an isolated individual. Even when only two people are physically present, ever-present others may include family members, loved ones, staff, clinicians, clergy, supervisors, commanders, and community members. The field also contains the influence of God, institution, tradition, law, memory, diagnosis, policy, and history.

The chaplain asks: Who is here without being here? Whose interests are being protected? Whose judgment is anticipated? Whose authority is being obeyed or resisted? Who is being spoken for, blamed, awaited, or mourned? An absent daughter may organize a treatment decision. A dead parent's judgment may govern a confession. A supervisor who is not present may constrain what staff can say. A congregation or command may shape what seems permissible. The chaplain need not interpret every absence, but cannot assume that only visible participants have roles.

TRAB-S is a way of looking at the chaplain's work in context. Gregory Bateson once called a role "one end of a relationship" and warned that one cannot study one end of a relationship and make sense. TRAB-S takes that warning seriously: task, role, authority, boundary, and soul are not separable properties but mutually defining relations. It has roots in the group relations work of Zachary Green and René Molenkamp, who named BART: Boundary, Authority, Role, and Task. BART has served well because it gives accessible language for observing group and organizational life. It helps us ask what contains the work, who has authority, what roles are being occupied, and what task is being pursued or avoided.

TRAB-S revises the order and deepens the frame: Task, Role, Authority, Boundary, and Soul.

Task comes first because no group or system exists without some task, even if the task is hidden, confused, avoided, or contested. A hospital unit has a task. A family around a dying person has a task. A prison has stated and unstated tasks. A military chaplain has tasks shaped by command, care, morale, conscience, and institutional mission. A CPE group has a learning task. A board has a governance task. When the task is unclear, everything else becomes unstable.

The clinical chaplain asks: What is the work here? What is the stated task? What is the hidden task? What task is being avoided? What task have I been asked to take up? Is the chaplain being invited into the real task or into a substitute task that protects the system from something harder?

Role follows task and embodies it, but no role exists alone: patient implies caregiver, chaplain implies a person or system being served, and leader implies those who authorize, follow, resist, or withdraw authority. Formal roles include patient, physician, nurse, chaplain, commander, inmate, officer, family spokesperson, supervisor, and trainee; informal roles include peacemaker, truth-teller, scapegoat, identified problem, good child, difficult family, spiritual one, rational one, and angry one. Roles distribute affect as care becomes nurturance, fear becomes watching, rage becomes challenge, or play becomes innovation. They are not simply assigned by job description; they are affect made social.

The clinical chaplain asks: What role am I in? What role am I being invited, assigned, seduced, or pressured into? What role is the patient carrying? What role has the family assigned to the physician, nurse, chaplain, God, institution, or an ever-present other? What role is forbidden?

Authority is the right, permission, burden, or fantasy of doing work on behalf of the group. Authority may be formal or informal. A physician has medical authority. A grandmother may have family authority. A chaplain may have symbolic authority. A patient may have moral authority. A staff member may hold practical authority because everyone trusts her. Authority can be projected onto someone who does not want it or withheld from someone who formally has it.

Authority channels affect as leaders absorb fear, contain rage, authorize care, and permit play. When authority fails, affect spreads uncontained: panic moves through a team, rage turns destructive, grief immobilizes, and cynicism protects against helplessness. The chaplain must notice where authority is located, how it is being used, and what feelings it is carrying.

Boundary is containment. Boundaries include time, space, role, confidentiality, ritual, discipline, tradition, chart, uniform, visiting hours, unit rules, command structure, prison walls, and the beginning and ending of encounters. Boundaries soothe fear when they are clear enough. They channel rage when they create fair process. They permit play when they make safety possible. Boundaries that are too porous allow affect to spill destructively. Boundaries that are too rigid deaden care.

Soul is the felt life of the system. Without soul, task, role, authority, and boundary become abstractions. A system is not only a structure. It is a network of consciousness. Each person brings a unique history that colors how feeling is activated. The systems themselves are shared enough to make recognition possible: fear, care, grief, rage, desire, play, and seeking move through groups as well as individuals.

TRAB-S is not a closed theory to impose on every encounter. It is a set of questions that helps the chaplain resist vagueness while remaining open to patterns the framework did not predict. A nurse asks for a chaplain because a family is "difficult." Task: what work is actually needed? Role: is the chaplain being asked to soothe, persuade, absorb rage, bless a decision, or take the family's side? Authority: who can decide what?

Boundary: what limits have collapsed? Soul: what fear, grief, guilt, or rage is moving through the system?

A prison chaplain is asked to speak with an inmate who is "manipulative." Task: pastoral care, security management, moral recognition, or staff relief? Role: chaplain, confessor, advocate, institutional agent, witness? Authority: what can the chaplain promise? Boundary: what must be confidential, reported, or clarified? Soul: what longing, rage, fear, shame, or seeking may be hiding inside the behavior named as manipulation?

A military chaplain is told morale is low. Task: morale maintenance, pastoral care, command consultation, ethical witness, grief work, or organizational diagnosis? Role: officer, chaplain, confidant, symbolic presence, critic, loyal servant? Authority: what belongs to command and what belongs to conscience? Boundary: what is private, privileged, operational, or communal? Soul: what grief, fear, loyalty, rage, care, or injury is animating the unit?

TRAB-S also protects the chaplain from self-deception. Chaplains often enter systems with a wish to help. But helping is not a task unless it is defined. A chaplain who does not understand task may take up whatever role the system offers. A chaplain who does not understand authority may overreach or abdicate. A chaplain who does not understand boundary may confuse intimacy with care. A chaplain who does not attend to soul may analyze structure while missing the living current of the encounter.

The Right Resource Model and TRAB-S belong together. Right Resource asks what kind of care is called for. TRAB-S asks what system is actually presenting. Together they help the chaplain avoid the two common failures: doing too little because chaplaincy is reduced to presence, and doing too much because chaplaincy is inflated into universal ministry.

The S is what prevents TRAB-S from becoming merely organizational. Soul here does not make the model pious. It makes it clinical. Task, role, authority, and boundary are always lived in feeling. A task may be clear on paper and intolerable in the body. A role may be formally assigned and affectively refused. Authority may be structurally legitimate and emotionally distrusted. A boundary may be well designed and still experienced as abandonment or control.

This is why systems work belongs in clinical chaplaincy. The chaplain is often invited into the affective residue of failed systems. A family calls because medicine has not contained fear. Staff call because policy has not contained moral distress. A prison asks the chaplain to calm what the institution has intensified. A military command asks for resilience when grief has not been mourned. TRAB-S helps the chaplain see that the presenting request may be only the visible edge of a system's affective life.

TRAB-S also keeps the chaplain from spiritualizing system problems. Not every anxiety is spiritual distress. Sometimes the task is unclear. Sometimes authority has failed. Sometimes the chaplain has been placed in an impossible role. Sometimes the boundary is wrong. Soul is always present, but soul does not erase structure.

In training, TRAB-S can be used after a case presentation. Instead of asking only what the chaplain felt or what the patient said, the group can ask: What was the task? What role did the chaplain take? What authority did the chaplain have or imagine? What boundary was tested? What soul-current moved through the encounter? This keeps case review from becoming either personal confession or technical critique. It places the chaplain inside a living system.

In institutional consultation, TRAB-S can prevent premature solutions. A leader may ask for a chaplaincy program because staff are burned out. Before designing an intervention, the consultant asks: What is the institution's task? What roles are staff being forced to occupy? Where has authority failed? What boundaries are being crossed? What grief, fear, rage, or moral injury is uncontained? Without these questions, chaplaincy may become another soothing resource applied to an unchanged system.

In supervision, TRAB-S helps the chaplain find the point of pressure. The question is not simply, "How did you feel?" It is, "Where did the system place you, and what did that evoke?" A chaplain who feels inexplicably helpless may have been assigned the role of powerless witness. A chaplain who feels grandiose may have been loaded with impossible authority. A chaplain who feels irritated by a family may be carrying staff rage. TRAB-S makes these possibilities discussable.

Practice Implications

> TRAB-S means Task, Role, Authority, Boundary, and Soul. It grows from BART but begins with task and grounds the system in felt life. The chaplain asks what work is required, what roles are being occupied, who has authority, what boundaries contain the work, and what affective current animates the system. TRAB-S is practical because it helps the chaplain know what is mine to do and what is not mine to do.

FIFTEEN
STAFF, TEAM, INSTITUTION

Clinical chaplaincy is not only patient care.

In healthcare this must be said plainly because chaplaincy is often measured through patient visits, referrals, deaths, rituals, and documentation. In prisons, military settings, schools, and public safety organizations, the equivalent measures may differ, but the distortion remains. Chaplaincy is reduced to direct service to individuals while the systems shaping those individuals remain unexamined.

The chaplain works with persons in systems. The chaplain also works with systems as systems.

Systems invite linear blame because blame simplifies anxiety. The problem becomes the patient, the family, the nurse, the physician, the chaplain, the leader, or the policy. Clinical perception asks instead how the parts are participating in a circular pattern of feedback. This does not erase responsibility. It locates responsibility within relationship and consequence rather than pretending that one isolated culprit explains the whole.

Staff distress is clinical material. A nurse who cannot enter a room after a traumatic death, a physician who becomes contemptuous toward a family, a guard who jokes cruelly after an inmate's suicide, a commander who speaks only in operational language after moral failure, a teacher who feels helpless before a student's despair - all may be presenting spiritual, moral, affective, and systemic distress. The chaplain's task is not merely to comfort them. It is to understand what the distress means and what resource is appropriate.

Moral distress is especially important. People suffer when they know or sense what should be done but feel unable to do it. Healthcare workers may continue treatments they believe are burdensome. Prison staff may enforce rules that feel dehumanizing. Military personnel may carry orders, memories, or actions that do not fit their moral identity. Institutional leaders may feel trapped between mission and finance. Chaplains often meet the residue of these conflicts.

The chaplain must avoid becoming the institution's emotional janitor. Institutions may use chaplains to absorb distress without changing conditions. A debriefing, prayer, blessing, or supportive conversation may be requested so that the system can return to function unchanged. Sometimes return to function is necessary. But clinical chaplaincy should not collude with avoidable harm by spiritualizing endurance.

The chaplain's unique domain on the interdisciplinary team must be clear. The chaplain is not the team's therapist, though therapeutic effects may occur. The chaplain is not the team's ethicist, though moral meaning may be central. The chaplain is not the team's social worker, though family systems matter. The chaplain is not the team's religious decorator, though ritual may be needed. The chaplain's domain is meaning, affect, relationship, and system as these bear upon soul.

This domain must be translated into team language. Teams need to know what chaplains see. A note saying "provided presence" rarely helps. A verbal report saying "family is anxious" may be too vague. A clinical chaplain might say, "The family appears to be using continued treatment to maintain a sense that they have not abandoned him. A direct recommendation without acknowledging that fear may intensify conflict." Or, "The patient's refusal of the plan seems less about information and more about loss of control after repeated institutional betrayals." Or, "Staff frustration is rising because the team is carrying unspoken grief after three similar deaths this week."

Such interpretive statements must be grounded, humble, and

useful. The chaplain should not perform insight. The chaplain should help the team care better.

Institutional leaders often wonder what to do with chaplains. Some see chaplains as necessary for accreditation, patient satisfaction, end-of-life care, religious accommodation, or staff support. Some value chaplains personally but cannot articulate their operational worth. Some reduce spiritual care to measurable interventions because measurement is the institutional language available. Chaplains sometimes respond defensively, insisting that their work is too sacred to measure. Both sides need better language.

A spiritual care service should be designed backward from the population's needs and the institution's intended aims. Its design should be ecological: differentiated resources, clear relationships, reliable feedback, and enough flexibility to respond when the actual need does not resemble the referral label. What forms of religious accommodation, spiritual distress care, serious-illness support, staff care, moral consultation, community connection, and high-acuity clinical work are actually required? What does the institution intend to improve, protect, or make possible? Staffing, training, referral pathways, and documentation should follow from those answers, not from inherited assumptions about what a chaplain customarily does.

Powell once put the institutional question with useful bluntness: when did chaplains last ask their non-chaplain colleagues when they most wanted—or believed they needed—a chaplain? The question does not let others define the whole profession. It forces chaplaincy to listen to the institution it claims to serve.

The Right Resource Model offers one bridge. Institutions should ask what spiritual care needs exist, at what level of acuity, and what resources are required. A high-functioning spiritual care system may include volunteers, community clergy, staff chaplains, psychodynamically informed clinical chaplains, educators, and consultants. The question is not whether chaplaincy is generally good. The question is whether the institution has the capability required by its population, staff, mission, and risks.

TRAB-S offers another bridge by asking what task the institution is pursuing, what role chaplaincy has been assigned, what authority it possesses, what boundaries protect or restrict the work, and what soul or affective life moves through the institution. Together these questions reveal whether chaplaincy is integrated, ornamental, overused, underused, or misused.

A hospital may say its task is healing while organizing around throughput. A prison may say its task is rehabilitation while organizing around control. A military command may say its task is mission while carrying unspoken grief. A school may say its task is education while functioning as containment for social despair. Chaplains who cannot read institutional contradiction will be used by it.

Staff care must also be distinguished from staff comfort. Staff sometimes need comfort. They also need spaces where grief, anger, shame, helplessness, and moral conflict can be named without being immediately managed away. Clinical chaplaincy can offer such spaces when properly authorized and boundaried. But staff care requires attention to role. Is the chaplain acting as peer, consultant, supervisor, ritual leader, debriefer, advocate, or confidential listener? Confusion of role can harm trust.

Confidentiality is complicated in systems work. Chaplains must understand institutional policy, legal requirements, ethical obligations, and the limits of confidentiality in their setting. They must not promise what they cannot keep. They must not conceal risk. They must not casually share intimate material in the name of team collaboration. Documentation and communication should serve care while respecting the person.

Confidentiality protects personal content; it does not require a secret method. Chaplains should be able to explain how referrals are triaged, what they assess, why an intervention was chosen, what they contribute to the plan of care, and when they refer elsewhere. The private details of an encounter may remain private while the discipline of the work remains visible. Demystifying chaplaincy helps institutions use it appropriately and keeps spiritual authority from becoming exemption from scrutiny.

The chaplain's authority with teams grows through reliability. Dramatic interventions rarely build trust. Clear observations, appropriate restraint, good referrals, accurate documentation, respect for other disciplines, and the capacity to remain thoughtful under pressure build authority over time. The chaplain who wants to be taken seriously must do serious work seriously.

The chaplain must also know when to challenge the team. Clinical collaboration does not mean compliance. If the team is dehumanizing a family, ignoring religious needs, misreading spiritual distress, using the chaplain to close a conflict, or avoiding moral truth, the chaplain may need to speak. The manner should be disciplined. The courage should be real.

Staff, team, and institution are not secondary to clinical chaplaincy; they are part of the field. Patients suffer within systems, families react to them, staff carry them, and leaders authorize them. The chaplain who sees only the person in the bed, cell, or office sees too little.

Practice Implications

> Clinical chaplaincy includes staff, teams, and institutions. Staff distress, moral injury, and institutional anxiety are clinical material. Chaplains should not become emotional janitors for systems that refuse change. The chaplain's unique team contribution is disciplined attention to meaning, affect, relationship, and system. Right Resource and TRAB-S help institutional leaders understand chaplaincy capability. Collaboration requires clarity, confidentiality, and courage.

SIXTEEN
CONTINUING FORMATION

Certification is not completion.

This may be one of the hardest truths for the profession to accept. Board certification can become a form of lifelong authorization. The chaplain has completed training, met standards, passed review, and entered professional status. From then on, much of the work may occur privately, behind closed doors, with minimal observation and little serious case review. Continuing education may be required, but continuing formation is not the same thing.

Clinical chaplaincy requires ongoing formation because the work continues to expose the chaplain. New settings, new populations, new losses, new institutional pressures, new personal stages of life, new cultural realities, and new theoretical developments all change the work. The chaplain who stops learning does not remain stable. The chaplain becomes habitual.

Bateson distinguished learning from learning to learn. Continuing formation requires both. A chaplain learns from a case, but also learns how the chaplain habitually frames cases, what differences are noticed, what contexts are excluded, and what kinds of correction can be tolerated.

Powell's phrasing—clinical pastoral training, education, and transformation—is useful here. Skill, understanding, and the formation of the practitioner belong together; none is finished at certification.

Case writing should continue after training. Almost no one does it. That is precisely why it matters.

A case study slows the work down. It requires sequence, memory, dialogue, observation, affect, self-reflection, formulation, and question. It reveals what the chaplain thought was happening and what may have been missed. It allows peers and supervisors to see the work. It makes the chaplain accountable to more than private conviction.

Raymond J. Lawrence belongs in this lineage as mentor, pioneer, and towering figure. His *Nine Clinical Cases* and *Nine More Clinical Cases* psychodynamically reinterpret cases first presented by Fitchett and Nolan. Their importance is not that they supply a diagnostic system to emulate, but that they model a return to reviewing a case, questioning its original formulation to see what another clinical reading discloses.

Case presentation is not humiliation but professional practice. Physicians present cases, psychotherapists seek consultation, analysts undergo supervision, social workers staff cases, and serious clinical professions review their work. Chaplaincy should not be exempt because the work is spiritual; if anything, its symbolic and intimate nature makes review more necessary.

No one should be the sole witness to the meaning of their own work.

Ongoing supervision should be normal after board certification. It may take different forms: individual supervision, peer consultation group, case conference, Balint-style group, group relations consultation, advanced clinical cohort, or periodic consultation with a trusted supervisor. The form matters less than the discipline. The chaplain must have a place to bring uncertainty, mistakes, attraction, shame, anger, boredom, failure, institutional pressure, and theological confusion.

A profession that treats supervision as remedial will remain clinically immature.

This is especially important because chaplaincy grants unusual access. Patients, families, prisoners, service members, students, and staff may disclose intimate material to a chaplain. They may assume confidentiality, wisdom, spiritual authority, or safety. Institutions may trust chaplains to move through vulnerable spaces with little observation. That trust is not a reason to avoid accountability. It is the reason accountability matters.

Continuing formation also requires reading. This is delicate because many chaplains do not read much and do not read long. The solution is not to abandon reading but to choose reading that matters. Clinical chaplains do not need to become scholars of everything. They need a living intellectual diet that deepens practice: Boisen, Pruyser, Lawrence, Powell, Cooper-White, Solms, Panksepp, Geertz, group relations, selected pastoral care classics, and serious case studies. Reading should return to practice. If it does not sharpen attention, deepen humility, or improve care, it is ornamental.

The individual learning contract should not end with CPE. Every chaplain should be able to name current learning edges: what is being avoided, which populations evoke judgment, what kinds of cases produce feelings of incompetence, which theories or rituals are overused, which boundaries are difficult, where authority is abdicated or inflated, and what changes in the field remain poorly understood.

Formation includes the body. Chaplaincy is embodied work. The chaplain carries stress, grief, vigilance, boredom, compassion, and institutional residue. Sleep, movement, spiritual practice, therapy, friendship, solitude, and pleasure are not luxuries. They affect clinical reliability. A depleted chaplain may still be kind, but depletion narrows perception and increases enactment.

Formation includes moral life. Chaplains should examine money, power, sexuality, ambition, resentment, envy, spiritual pride, and institutional compromise. Chaplaincy provides many opportunities for hidden gratification: being needed, being trusted, being special, being spiritually superior, being the one who understands. These gratifications are not shameful because they occur. They become dangerous when they remain unexamined.

Continuing formation also includes limits. A chaplain cannot read everything, serve everyone, master every tradition, respond to every crisis, or carry every grief. Formation includes learning what is not mine. It includes referral, collaboration, sabbath, and relinquishment.

A mature clinical chaplain remains not vaguely humble but actually teachable: able to say, 'I used to see it this way; now I am beginning to see it differently,' willing to present a case, be wrong, change practice, hear that a beloved intervention may be self-serving, discover that a patient experienced the encounter differently, and let the field advance.

The profession needs this more than it needs more slogans. It needs chaplains who continue to submit their work to reflection, not because they are weak, but because the work is strong medicine.

Peer review after certification will require cultural change. Many chaplains have learned to associate case presentation with student status. Once certified, they may feel that presenting cases exposes inadequacy. The opposite is true. The capacity to present one's work for review is a sign of professional maturity. A chaplain who cannot bear scrutiny is not safer because the work remains private.

Case review should include successful encounters as well as failures, because good work also needs examination. What made it good, what did the chaplain notice or restrain, what hypothesis changed, what resource was rightly engaged, and what boundary held? Without reviewing good work, a profession cannot teach excellence; without reviewing failed or uncertain work, it cannot become honest.

Supervision also protects the chaplain from isolation. The work can be lonely precisely because it is intimate. Chaplains often hear what others do not hear and then carry it alone. A peer or supervisor does not remove the burden, but helps metabolize it. The soul of the chaplain is one of the instruments of care. Instruments require tending.

Practice Implications

> Certification is not completion. Continuing education is not the same as continuing formation. Case writing and peer review should continue after training. Ongoing supervision should be normal, not remedial. Reading must deepen practice. The chaplain's body, moral life, and limits are part of clinical reliability.

SEVENTEEN
THE FUTURE OF CHAPLAINCY

The future of chaplaincy will not be secured by nostalgia.

It will not be secured by insisting that institutions should value chaplains because chaplains are kind, spiritual, traditional, inclusive, or comforting. It will not be secured by replacing religious language with generic spiritual care language and hoping the field thereby becomes more acceptable. It will not be secured by certification alone. It will not be secured by research metrics alone. It will not be secured by chaplains becoming amateur therapists, ritual generalists, or institutional empaths.

The future of chaplaincy depends on clarity of capability.

What can chaplains do that matters? What kinds of chaplains are needed for what kinds of situations? What training forms those chaplains? What level of acuity requires what resource? What does clinical chaplaincy contribute to persons and systems that is not otherwise supplied? These questions cannot be answered with slogans.

The field has often confused coverage with capability. Coverage asks whether a chaplain is present, available, and responsive. Capability asks whether the right resource is available for the actual need. Coverage can be scheduled. Capability must be formed. Coverage is necessary in many institutions. Capability is what makes coverage worth having.

Chaplains who fear for their jobs may understandably experience higher expectations as a threat. But the greater threat is a role so indistinct that institutions cannot say what competence they are retaining. Raising the bar makes chaplains more—not less—valuable when it produces demonstrable capability: better assessment, clearer documentation, wiser referral, stronger collaboration, more reliable high-acuity care, and accountable consultation. Advanced formation does not guarantee employment. It gives institutions a clearer reason to retain and invest in chaplaincy.

An Ecology of Clinical Chaplaincy

The future requires a differentiated ecology of spiritual care. Volunteers, community clergy, professional chaplains, clinical chaplains, psychodynamically informed chaplains, educators, consultants, and institutional leaders all have possible roles. The problem is not that one role exists. The problem is when roles are blurred, inflated, or used interchangeably. A healthy field should be able to say what each resource can and cannot do.

This will require courage from chaplains. They must stop claiming everything spiritual as their domain while complaining that no one understands their work; stop hiding behind presence when clinical formulation is required; stop performing rituals for which they have no authority; stop accepting marginality as identity; and stop imagining that being liked is the same as being clinically useful.

It will also require courage from institutions. Institutions must stop using chaplains as low-cost emotional absorbers. They must stop calling chaplains only when the real problem has already escalated. They must stop measuring spiritual care only by activity counts. They must recognize that serious chaplaincy requires training, supervision, staffing, authority, and integration.

The future requires a renewed Boisenian seriousness. Boisen's original intuition was radical: learn from living human documents; bring theology into disciplined relationship with the human sciences; train through supervised encounter with actual persons in crisis; take the inner world seriously. That intuition remains unfinished. It must now be brought into conversation with contemporary psychodynamic thought, affective neuroscience, neuropsychoanalysis, interpretive anthropology, group relations, and institutional realities.

This renewal should not be antiquarian. Boisen is not important because he is an ancestor to be honored. He is important because his method still points forward. The living human document is not exhausted. In a post-denominational, plural, anxious, and institutionally complex world, the need to read persons and systems with depth is greater, not less.

The future also requires better writing and teaching. Chaplains often do not read much and do not read long. This is not an insult; it is a professional reality. The field is busy, emotionally burdened, and often underformed intellectually. Therefore, the books and materials that matter must be clear, lean, practical, and serious. They should not be shallow. They should be readable enough to be used.

A future-oriented chaplaincy needs small, durable conceptual tools: Right Resource Model, fourfold clinical lens, cues and clues, clinical chaplaincy diagnosis, spirituality and religion after religion, non-offering stance toward prayer and ritual, TRAB-S, ongoing case review. These tools can travel across healthcare, prisons, military, schools, and other settings because they are not tied to one institutional form. They are ways of perceiving human systems under pressure.

No one of these tools is the architecture of the whole. Together they form a working ecology of clinical chaplaincy. Each directs attention to relations the others might miss. Each remains incomplete without the others. Their value lies not in closing the system but in helping clinicians move among levels: person and culture, body and symbol, dyad and institution, stated task and unconscious task, immediate crisis and longer history.

The future of chaplaincy also depends on formation communities. No single book can make a clinical chaplain. No weekend seminar can do it. No certification board can guarantee it. Clinical chaplaincy requires communities of practice where cases are presented, supervisors supervise, peers challenge, theory is tested, and chaplains remain accountable. The field needs more than credentials. It needs disciplined fellowships, cohorts, case conferences, and consultation groups.

There is also a public task. Chaplaincy must explain itself to institutional leaders without surrendering its soul. Leaders need language for staffing, acuity, outcomes, risk, staff support, patient experience, moral distress, and resource allocation. Chaplains need language for meaning, affect, relationship, system, ritual, religion, and soul. The future belongs to those who can translate without reduction.

The future will also require chaplains to work beyond healthcare without losing clinical rigor. Prisons need chaplains who understand shame, violence, institutional control, religious identity, and redemption without becoming agents of the system's denial. The military needs chaplains who understand moral injury, authority, loyalty, grief, and mission without becoming merely morale officers. Schools need chaplains or spiritual care leaders who understand anxiety, identity, belonging, family systems, and the sacredness of becoming. First-responder settings need chaplains who understand trauma, humor, silence, loyalty, and the ritual life of those who meet catastrophe professionally.

Healthcare remains central, but it should not define the whole field.

The future of chaplaincy is not the disappearance of religion. Nor is it the restoration of a prior religious order. It is the disciplined care of souls in a world where soul speaks many languages. Some of those languages are ancient. Some are improvised. Some are secular. Some are embodied in food, fitness, politics, recovery, family, nation, profession, or silence. The clinical chaplain must learn to hear without forcing translation too quickly.

The field will mature when it can hold several truths at once: chaplaincy is ancient; chaplaincy is changing; spiritual care is broad; clinical chaplaincy is specialized; presence matters; presence is not enough; religion persists; religion moves; institutions need chaplains; institutions also misuse chaplains; certification matters; formation must continue.

The future of chaplaincy is not guaranteed. It must be formed.

The future belongs to a chaplaincy that can be both deep and clear, structured and open, clinically accountable and capable of surprise. It belongs to chaplains who can perceive differently so that meaning and purpose may emerge where crisis has made the world unrecognizable.

Practice Implications

The future of chaplaincy depends on clarity of capability, not nostalgia or generic spiritual care language. Coverage must be distinguished from capability. The field needs differentiated resources and serious formation communities. Chaplaincy must translate its value to institutions without reducing its work to metrics. The principles in this book should travel beyond healthcare into prisons, military, schools, public safety, and other systems under pressure.

AFTERWORD: THE WORK BEFORE US

Clinical chaplaincy stands at a threshold.

The field can continue as it is: valued by some, misunderstood by many, often thinly described, sometimes deeply practiced, frequently underused, occasionally overextended, and too often content with language that does not match the depth of the work. Or it can become clearer.

Clarity will require distinctions. Spiritual care is broader than clinical chaplaincy, professional chaplaincy is broader than psychodynamically informed clinical chaplaincy, and supportive presence is not the same as clinical practice. Ritual support is not ritual authority, cultural humility is not cultural omniscience, and chaplaincy is not therapy even though it is not less than clinical. Certification is not completion, just as coverage is not capability.

Clarity will also require courage. Chaplains must stop accepting roles that flatter and diminish them. Institutions must stop treating chaplains as generic comfort providers. Training programs must stop confusing exposure with formation. Supervisors must form clinicians who can think, feel, interpret, and act. Professional bodies must make room for levels of competence and acuity. Chaplains must submit their work to review.

This book has argued for clinical chaplaincy as the disciplined practice of perceiving differently so that meaning and purpose can emerge in the midst of crisis, distress, loss, grief, or perplexity. Meaning, affect, relationship, and system form the fourfold ecology through which that perception is trained in the recovery of soul. Meaning asks what world is at stake. Affect asks what feeling is moving the person or system. Relationship asks what is happening between persons, roles, histories, and internal objects. System asks what task, role, authority, boundary, and institutional field shape the encounter. Soul names the felt life that makes all this matter.

The work is ancient and contemporary. Ancient, because the care of souls long predates modern professions. Contemporary, because the worlds in which souls suffer have changed. The chaplain now meets persons for whom religion may be church, mosque, synagogue, temple, scripture, sacrament, nature, CrossFit, food purity, recovery, nation, identity, family, science, medicine, or nothing that will accept the name religion. The chaplain meets systems that speak in metrics, policies, security, command, throughput, liability, and outcomes. The chaplain must learn to hear soul there too.

The clinical chaplain asks what is really going on and what is trying to become meaningful before deciding what it means. The chaplain then asks what care is called for, what belongs or does not belong to the role, and what is being felt, defended, held sacred, or threatened. The final questions are systemic and practical: what pattern connects the persons, affects, symbols, roles, and systems; what role is being assigned; what resource is right; and what must be spoken or left in silence?

These questions do not make chaplaincy less spiritual. They make it more honest.

The recovery of soul is not the chaplain's possession. It is the work of persons and communities struggling to remain alive to meaning under pressure. The clinical chaplain's privilege is to serve that work with humility, discipline, courage, and love.

This book is complete only when it returns the reader to the field. The next patient, family, team, institution, or community will not repeat the last. The principles remain; the pattern changes. The work before us is to look again.

A NOTE ON TRAINING

This book implies the need for a reform of training. Clinical chaplains are not formed by exposure alone. They require psychodynamic and systems learning, disciplined use of self, supervised practice, sustained case writing and review, and communities in which work continues to be shared and consulted after certification.

ClinicalChaplaincy.org is an effort in support of that kind of formation through teaching, supervision, case-based learning, and continuing professional development opportunities. It is named here not as the sole owner of this argument or the exclusive answer to the field. The need belongs to chaplaincy as a whole. Programs should be judged by the quality of their formation, the accountability of their practice, and the capabilities those they have trained can demonstrate.

APPENDIX A. KEY TERMS AND WORKING DEFINITIONS

This lexicon defines terms as they are used in this book. It is designed for readers who may have little prior exposure to psychodynamic thought, affective neuroscience, anthropology, semiotics, or group relations. These are working definitions rather than exhaustive scholarly accounts. They should make the manuscript usable without pretending to replace the traditions from which the terms come.

Abduction

Abduction is the disciplined formation of a plausible hypothesis from incomplete signs. Unlike deduction, it does not prove a conclusion, and unlike simple induction, it is not merely a summary of repeated observations. The chaplain notices cues and clues, asks what account best fits them, tests that account gently, and remains ready to revise it.

Acuity

Acuity is the urgency, depth, complexity, and risk of a need. It is not the same as visible intensity: a quiet person may be in high-acuity spiritual distress, while an emotionally expressive person may not require specialized clinical care. Acuity helps determine the right resource, timing, and level of follow-up.

Affect

Affect is the felt dimension of experience: emotion, mood, bodily tone, urgency, pleasure, pain, dread, longing, anger, tenderness, excitement, or numbness. Affect often organizes perception and action before a person can explain what is happening. In this book, feeling is not secondary data; it is part of the ground of consciousness and meaning.

Authority

Authority is the right to do work. Formal or delegated authority comes from an office, institution, policy, group, supervisor, or religious tradition. Personal authority is the capacity to take up work responsibly from one's formation, judgment, and integrity. Authority entails responsibility and accountability and should be accompanied by the tools and resources required for the task.

BART

BART means Boundary, Authority, Role, and Task. In group relations it is a practical framework for observing structural and unconscious dynamics in groups and organizations. It is a useful partial lens, not a complete theory of human systems. TRAB-S reorders and extends it for clinical chaplaincy.

Boundary

A boundary is a container for work. Boundaries may involve time, task, territory, role, responsibility, resources, confidentiality, body, ritual authority, tradition, or policy. Useful boundaries are clear enough to hold the task and flexible enough to permit thought, care, and transition; boundaries that are too porous spill anxiety, while boundaries that are too rigid may deaden the work.

Chaplain

A chaplain is someone who does ministry outside an ordinary congregational setting. The term identifies a broad role and location of service; it does not by itself specify training, credential, method, authority, or competence.

Chart Note and Case Writing

A chart note is a concise clinical communication to the care team: what was assessed, what was done, what changed, and what continuity is needed. Case writing is a fuller educational account used for supervision, consultation, and formation. Confusing the two either overloads the record or starves learning. Responsible charting helps establish the chaplain as an accountable member of the clinical team.

Clinical Chaplaincy

Clinical chaplaincy is the disciplined practice of perceiving persons and human systems differently so that meaning and purpose can emerge in the midst of crisis, distress, loss, grief, or perplexity. It proceeds through observation, provisional formulation, intervention or restraint, documentation when appropriate, consultation, case review, and continuing formation. It is clinical because of method, not merely because of setting or credential.

Clinical Chaplaincy Diagnosis

Clinical chaplaincy diagnosis is not medical or psychiatric diagnosis. It is the disciplined, provisional formulation of what is spiritually, religiously, morally, symbolically, affectively, relationally, and systemically at stake. It asks what is really going on in the domain of chaplaincy care and what kind of response or resource is called for.

Clinical Cycle

The clinical cycle is notice, formulate, test, intervene, document, reflect, and revise. It is recursive rather than linear: an intervention produces new information, and reflection should change subsequent perception and practice. The cycle disciplines intuition without pretending that care can be reduced to a sequence of techniques.

Clinical Formulation

A clinical formulation is a concise, provisional account of what may be happening and why. It links observations with affect, meaning, relationship, history, symbols, system pressure, and resource fit. A formulation is not a label attached to a person; it is a hypothesis made useful by the care it helps the chaplain consider and by its openness to revision.

Containment

Containment is the capacity of a person, relationship, group, or institution to hold difficult affect long enough for it to be experienced and thought about without being immediately evacuated, acted out, or passed to someone else. Containment is not suppression. It gives feeling a form in which meaning and choice may become possible.

Context

Context is the network of relationships and conditions within which a word, action, symbol, symptom, role, or event becomes meaningful. Context is not background added after the fact. It is part of the phenomenon being understood.

Countertransference

Countertransference refers to the chaplain's conscious and unconscious responses to a person or system. Those responses arise from the chaplain's own history and from what is being communicated in the present relationship. They are clinical data, not automatic truth. They require reflection, boundaries, consultation, and humility.

Cues and Clues

Cues are observable signals that draw attention; clues are cues considered for what they may indicate. Tone, silence, gesture, contradiction, an object in the room, a staff comment, or the chaplain's internal response may become a clue. Neither cues nor clues interpret themselves. Their meaning is contextual and must be tested.

Defense

A defense is a way a person or system protects itself from affect, conflict, knowledge, or vulnerability that feels difficult to bear. Defenses may be adaptive, costly, or both. They are not moral defects to be exposed. Clinical care asks what a defense protects and whether another way of bearing the experience is becoming possible.

Displacement

Displacement occurs when feeling attached to one person, event, or conflict is redirected toward a safer or more available target. Anger at illness may be directed at staff; grief may appear as a complaint about parking; institutional anxiety may be deposited in the chaplain. The apparent target is real, but it may not be the whole source.

Ecological Perception

Ecological perception attends to persons, affects, symbols, relationships, and systems as mutually shaping rather than isolated. It asks what context gives an event meaning, what pattern connects the parts, what feedback sustains the pattern, and how the observer participates in the field.

Enactment

An enactment is a relational pattern communicated and created in interaction rather than stated directly. A patient, family, team, and chaplain may find themselves doing together what no one can yet say—for example, rescuing, abandoning, blaming, controlling, or becoming helpless. Recognition of enactment can restore thought and choice.

Ever-Present Others

Ever-present others are persons not physically present whose interests, needs, authority, memory, anticipated response, or symbolic significance actively shape an encounter. They may be named—family members, clinicians, clergy, supervisors, commanders, or community members—or present unconsciously as internalized figures or imagined audiences. The term does not make every absence clinically significant. It directs the chaplain to ask who is being represented, protected, obeyed, resisted, spoken for, awaited, or mourned.

Field

The field is the total relational, emotional, symbolic, bodily, and institutional situation in which an encounter occurs. It includes those physically present, ever-present others whose interests or impact are active in it, and the larger systems that give the encounter its setting. The chaplain does not stand outside it. What the chaplain feels, wants, avoids, or is invited to become may be part of the field, though it must never be treated as self-validating evidence.

Group Relations

Group relations is an experiential tradition for studying conscious and unconscious life in groups and organizations. Associated with Bion, Tavistock, A. K. Rice, and related work, it treats participation itself as a source of learning about task, authority, role, boundary, leadership, anxiety, and off-task behavior.

Interfaith Chaplaincy

Interfaith chaplaincy is disciplined care across differences of religion, spirituality, culture, and symbolic world. It does not mean that one chaplain possesses every tradition or is authorized to perform every rite. Competence includes curiosity, cultural humility, knowledge of limits, careful referral, and respect for the authority of communities and tradition-specific representatives.

Intersubjectivity

Intersubjectivity names the fact that experience is formed between subjects as well as within them. A clinical encounter is neither wholly the patient's interior event nor the chaplain's detached observation. Each person affects and is affected by the other, and understanding develops in that relational field.

Intervention and Restraint

An intervention is any deliberate clinical action, including a question, reflection, silence, prayer, ritual, referral, boundary, chart note, or team communication. Restraint is also a clinical act when the chaplain chooses not to interpret, offer ritual, seek closure, or take up an unauthorized role. The question is not whether the chaplain did something visible, but whether the response fit.

Living Human Document

The living human document is Boisen's phrase for the person whose life, crisis, history, religious experience, distress, and meaning-making become the text of clinical inquiry. The phrase is powerful, but it must be used humbly. Persons are not documents written for the chaplain, and every reading is partial.

Meaning and Meaning-World

Meaning is not merely an explanation applied to experience. It is the organization by which a world holds together and action becomes possible. A meaning-world is the lived network of stories, loyalties, symbols, expectations, practices, authorities, and hopes through which reality comes to feel coherent and uniquely real.

Memory Trace

A memory trace is the persistence of past experience in present feeling, bodily readiness, expectation, image, or relational pattern, whether or not the person can narrate an explicit memory. Clinical chaplaincy may work with the effects of such traces without trying to force hidden material into conscious recollection.

Ministry

Ministry is intentional service undertaken from a religious, spiritual, or meaning-bearing vocation. In this book the word does not itself guarantee clinical method, institutional authority, or competence.

Negative Capability

Negative capability is the capacity to remain with uncertainty, ambiguity, and mystery without rushing into premature explanation or action. In chaplaincy it permits the honest position, "I do not yet know," while attention continues. It is not passivity; it is disciplined tolerance of not knowing.

Non-Offering Stance

The non-offering stance is the discipline of not making the chaplain's ritual repertoire the menu. It does not mean withholding care. It allows prayer, ritual, blessing, silence, and symbolic action to emerge from the person's world, the clinical situation, consent, and appropriate authority rather than from the chaplain's need to perform closure.

Participant Observer

A participant observer takes part in a human situation while also examining what is happening and how their own participation affects it. Chaplains are always participants in the clinical field. The discipline lies in using that involvement as data without imagining either complete detachment or complete identification.

Pastoral Diagnosis

Pastoral diagnosis is the earlier language, associated especially with Paul Pruyser, for disciplined discernment of the religious and pastoral dimensions of a person's situation. This book uses clinical chaplaincy diagnosis to emphasize setting-transcending method, provisional formulation, and resource fit while remaining in continuity with that tradition.

Pattern

A pattern is an organization of differences and relationships that recurs or holds a system together. Clinical attention looks for pattern without assuming that recurrence makes the pattern fixed, that the pattern belongs to one individual, or that noticing a pattern explains everything.

Prediction Error

Prediction error is the mismatch between what we implicitly expect and what occurs. When consequential, it increases uncertainty and may be registered as affective arousal, prompting defense, action, or revision of the model through which experience is organized. In clinical chaplaincy, prediction error helps explain why crisis may unsettle meaning, relationship, and bodily equilibrium at once.

Presence

Presence is disciplined availability to the person and system before the chaplain. It may be necessary, but it is not sufficient. Presence becomes clinical when it includes attention, restraint, formulation, timing, accountability, and fit.

Primary Emotional Systems

Primary emotional systems are evolutionarily conserved affective-motivational systems identified through cross-species affective neuroscience and used here as aids to clinical attention. They are the empirically grounded successors to, but not exact equivalents of, the older psychoanalytic drive concept. SEEKING concerns exploration, wanting, pursuit, and possibility; CARE, nurturance, attachment, and protection; PLAY, joy, experiment, flexibility, and reciprocity; LUST, sexual and erotic desire; RAGE, protest when need or movement is blocked; FEAR, threat, danger, avoidance, and protection; and PANIC/GRIEF, separation distress, loss, abandonment, and longing for reunion. The seven do not constitute a complete catalogue of human emotion: complex emotions such as shame and guilt join primary affect with learning, memory, relationship, and thought. The terms are questions for listening, not labels to impose on persons.

Prior

In predictive processing, a prior is an expectation the brain–mind brings to present experience before all the current evidence has been taken in. Priors are not necessarily conscious beliefs. They arise from bodily need, memory, attachment, repeated experience, culture, religion, and other symbolic systems. They shape what we notice and anticipate; prediction error occurs when experience consequentially departs from them.

Professional Chaplain

A professional chaplain makes chaplaincy a profession, often with formal education, clinical training, certification, institutional employment, and accountability to professional standards. Professional chaplaincy and clinical chaplaincy overlap, but they are not identical; professional status alone does not establish advanced psychodynamic or systems competence.

Projection

Projection is the attribution to another person or group of a feeling, wish, fear, motive, or expectation that is difficult to recognize as one's own. The projected material may still fit something real in the other person. The clinical task is not to declare projection but to examine how inner and outer reality are being organized together.

Projective Identification

Projective identification is an interpersonal process in which a feeling or role is not only attributed to another person but communicated in a way that may pressure the other to feel or enact it. A chaplain may suddenly feel helpless, rescuing, punitive, or uniquely necessary. The experience may be informative, but it must be reflected on and tested rather than presumed to reveal another person's unconscious.

Psychodynamic

Psychodynamic refers to attention to the forces that move mental and relational life, including conscious and unconscious motivation, affect, defense, conflict, memory, repetition, transference, and the presence of the past in the present. Psychodynamically informed chaplaincy is not psychotherapy in clerical dress. It uses these forms of attention within the chaplain's task, role, authority, boundaries, and time.

Purpose

Purpose is the forward-directed dimension of meaning: the aims, commitments, relationships, or desired states that organize action and make continued effort feel worthwhile. Meaning helps make experience intelligible; purpose helps answer, 'Given this, toward what can I now move?' In crisis, purpose may contract from a comprehensive life project to the next faithful, loving, necessary, or survivable act.

Rationalization

Rationalization is a plausible explanation that protects a person or system from a more difficult motive, conflict, or feeling. The explanation may contain truth. Its clinical significance lies in what it organizes, permits, or avoids, not in whether the chaplain can expose it as false.

Reflexivity

Reflexivity is disciplined examination of how the observer's history, identity, authority, body, assumptions, and desires shape perception and action. It is more than self-awareness. Reflexivity asks how the chaplain is participating in what is being observed and how that participation should alter the work.

Religion and Spirituality

Religion and spirituality are not simply identical, but neither are they clinical opposites. Spirituality may name a symbolic and meaning-bearing life without formal institutional affiliation; religion may name a more explicitly communal, traditional, or organized system. Following Geertz, both can be examined as systems of symbols that establish powerful moods and motivations and make an order of existence feel uniquely real.

Religious Function

Religious function is the work a practice, object, community, story, discipline, or institution performs when it organizes a general order of existence and carries sacred weight. It may appear in a named religion, but also in recovery, health, fitness, nation, family, work, ecology, or identity. The label is less important than what gives life meaning, obligation, hope, taboo, belonging, or salvation.

Right Resource Model

The Right Resource Model of Spiritual/Pastoral Care is a collaborative acuity-competency model. It asks who needs what, from whom, at what depth, and toward what end. It aligns need, acuity, competence, authority, available resources, referral, and review so that neither a generic chaplain nor any other single resource is expected to provide every form of care.

Role

Role is the way task is embodied in a person or position. Formal roles are conferred through position, credential, or explicit assignment; informal roles emerge in the life of a relationship or system. A role may be assigned, ascribed, invited, or taken up. Clinical attention asks how the role relates to task, authority, boundary, and the person's valence.

Semiotics

Semiotics is the study of signs and how meaning is made. Clinical chaplaincy is semiotic because it attends to words, gestures, silences, images, objects, rituals, symptoms, absences, and relationships as possible signs. A sign has no useful clinical meaning apart from context and interpretation.

Sign: Icon, Index, and Symbol

An icon signifies through resemblance, as a portrait resembles a person. An index signifies through an actual connection, as smoke indicates fire or a trembling hand indicates arousal. A symbol signifies through learned convention, as a flag, sacrament, diagnosis, team logo, or wedding ring does. In lived experience one sign may function in more than one way.

Soul

Soul names the felt aliveness of a person or system. The term may carry metaphysical meanings when those meanings belong to the person before us, but this book does not require agreement about them. Clinically, soul refers to consciousness and subjectivity attached to affect, memory, meaning, and relationship—the lived sense that something matters.

Spiritual Care

Spiritual care names the broad domain of attention to meaning, purpose, sacredness, connection, hope, identity, value, and ultimate concern. It may be offered by patients themselves, loved ones, communities, nurses, physicians, social workers, volunteers, clergy, ritual specialists, chaplains, and others. Clinical chaplaincy names one disciplined method within that larger field.

Spiritual Distress and Impaired Religiosity

Spiritual distress is disruption in a person's capacity to experience or integrate meaning, purpose, hope, connection, or transcendence. Impaired religiosity is difficulty relying on or participating in the beliefs, practices, rituals, obligations, or community that ordinarily support religious life. The two may overlap, but neither should be inferred from affiliation, nonaffiliation, or a single screening answer.

Symbolic World

A symbolic world is the lived network of meanings, loyalties, practices, prohibitions, memories, authorities, and hopes through which a person or group experiences reality as meaningful. A named religion may be one symbolic world. So may recovery, military service, family, health, nation, body practice, ecology, or work.

System

A system is a living organization of persons, roles, relationships, rules, histories, boundaries, resources, feedback, and task. A family, care team, congregation, department, institution, or society may be considered as a system. A systemic view asks how the parts mutually shape one another and what the whole appears organized to preserve or accomplish.

Task

Task is the work a person, group, or institution has gathered to do. The primary task is the intended work; the survival task preserves the person or system; the process task is work required to become able to do the primary task. Tasks are dynamic and affective. What a system says its task is may differ from what its behavior reveals.

Thick Description

Thick description interprets an act within the layers of context, convention, relationship, history, and meaning that make it intelligible. A blink and a wink may involve the same movement but are not the same act. Clinical chaplaincy requires enough contextual description to know what kind of event is actually occurring.

TRAB-S

TRAB-S means Task, Role, Authority, Boundary, and Soul. It grows from BART but begins with the work, then asks how the work is embodied, authorized, and contained. Soul names the felt life that animates all four. The framework helps a chaplain ask what is mine to do, what is not mine to do, and what feeling is organizing the system.

Transference

Transference is the carrying of feelings, expectations, fears, wishes, and relational patterns from earlier relationships into a present one. A chaplain may be experienced as parent, judge, rescuer, betrayer, priest, authority, or hoped-for protector beyond anything the chaplain has intentionally done. Transference is ordinary relational life, not proof of pathology.

Unconscious

The unconscious refers to mental, relational, and systemic processes outside immediate awareness that nevertheless shape feeling, perception, memory, behavior, and role. It is not merely a locked room of secrets waiting for the chaplain to expose. Clinical work often addresses its effects by noticing pattern and relationship without trying to make everything conscious.

Use of Self

Use of self is the disciplined employment of the chaplain's perception, affective response, history, authority, body, and relational presence in the service of care. It requires reflexivity, boundaries, consultation, and continuing supervision. It is not unprocessed self-expression or permission to make the encounter about the chaplain.

Valence

Valence is a person's recurring tendency to take up certain roles in a group, especially under anxiety. One person may reliably become rescuer, challenger, dependent member, peacemaker, skeptic, or bearer of grief. Valence is shaped by affect and history but is not destiny. Recognizing it can increase freedom not to enact the familiar role automatically.

APPENDIX B. TRAB-S: A WORKING GUIDE

TRAB-S is a framework for reading human systems, not a checklist and not a total theory. It grows from Green and Molenkamp's BART—Boundary, Authority, Role, and Task—but begins with Task because role, authority, and boundary make sense only in relation to work. It adds Soul because no human system is merely structural. Every task, role, authority, and boundary is lived in feeling.

The summaries below provide a working meaning for each rubric. The questions are examples, not a script. In practice, one good question may open more than a completed inventory.

Task

Task is the work a person, group, or institution has gathered to do. The primary task names the intended work. The survival task is the work of preserving the person or system itself. The process task is the work required before the primary task can be done. These tasks are dynamic. Under anxiety, the stated task may be displaced by avoidance, dependency, fight or flight, pairing, oneness, or activity that looks productive while protecting the system from its actual work. In TRAB-S, task is always affective: it matters what the work feels like and what feelings it mobilizes.

Questions one might ask:

- What is the stated or primary task here? Who has defined it?
- What survival task is competing with the primary task—for the patient, family, staff, chaplain, or institution?
- What process work must occur before the primary task can be taken up?
- What does the system appear organized to do, regardless of what it says it is doing?
- What task has the chaplain actually been asked to serve? Is that the real task, a displaced task, or an invitation to help avoid the task?
- What feelings does the task evoke, and how are those feelings helping or obstructing the work?

Role

Role is how task is embodied. A formal role is conferred through position, credential, job description, tradition, or explicit assignment. Informal roles emerge in relationship and may be assigned, ascribed, invited, or taken up without anyone naming them. People also bring valence—a recurring tendency to occupy certain roles under pressure. Role is therefore more than title. It is affect made social, and it may either support the task or become the way a system avoids it.

Questions one might ask:

- What is my formal role, and what does that role authorize me to do?
- What informal role am I being invited to occupy? What role have I already taken?
- How do the patient, family, staff, and institution appear to understand the chaplain's role?
- Who is carrying the roles of rescuer, expert, problem, victim,

challenger, peacemaker, believer, rational one, angry one, or silent one?

- Which ever-present others are shaping the work, and whose interests, needs, judgment, or authority is someone in the room carrying?
- Are multiple roles in conflict—for example, staff supporter, patient advocate, religious functionary, clinician, and institutional representative?
- What is my valence in this situation? Which familiar role makes me feel useful, safe, admired, or necessary?

Authority

Authority is the right to do work. Formal or delegated authority comes from a person, group, institution, office, policy, or tradition. Personal authority is the capacity to take up work responsibly from one's formation, judgment, and integrity. Authorization entails responsibility and accountability; it should also be accompanied by the time, information, access, supervision, and other resources needed to perform the task. Authority may be conferred, taken up, abdicated, exceeded, attacked, or projected. In TRAB-S, authority also channels collective affect: it may contain fear and rage, authorize care and play, or permit grief to be acknowledged.

Questions one might ask:

- Who has formal authority to define the task, make a decision, allocate a resource, or call a boundary?
- What authority belongs to the chaplain's institutional role, clinical formation, and religious or spiritual tradition—and what does not?
- Has the authority required for this work been clearly delegated and understood?
- Do the people charged with the task have the tools, access, time, information, and support needed to carry it out?
- Where is authority being taken up, abdicated, exceeded, attacked, or projected onto someone else?

- Who will be responsible and accountable for what is decided or done?

Boundary

Boundary is the container for work. Time, task, territory, role, responsibility, resources, confidentiality, tradition, ritual, and institutional policy may all create boundaries. Useful boundaries are clearly specified, sufficiently agreed upon, and reliably observed. They may also be understood as regions of transition rather than lines without thickness: admission and discharge, referral and handoff, entering and leaving a room, or moving from one role to another. Boundaries should serve the task. A porous boundary may spill anxiety into the system; a rigid one may deaden care, thought, and play.

Questions one might ask:

- What boundaries contain this work: time, task, place, role, confidentiality, ritual authority, body, family, team, record, policy, or resources?
- Are the relevant boundaries clear, agreed upon, and observed?
- Which boundaries are too porous, and what anxiety or responsibility is spilling across them?
- Which boundaries are too rigid, and what care, thought, grief, or play is being prevented?
- What transition or handoff needs deliberate attention?
- What boundary must the chaplain hold, and what boundary might the chaplain be tempted to cross in order to feel useful?

Soul

Soul names the felt aliveness of a person or system—the lived fact of consciousness and subjectivity. It is not a fifth box to be considered after the structural work is complete. It is what makes task matter, role attractive or burdensome, authority reassuring or threatening, and boundary containing or suffocating. SEEKING, CARE, PLAY, LUST, RAGE, FEAR, and PANIC/GRIEF animate the whole system. Naming Soul prevents TRAB-S from becoming organizational machinery and returns attention to what is felt, sacred, threatened, defended, desired, and grieved.

Questions one might ask:

- What is the felt life of this person, family, team, or institution?
- Which primary emotional systems appear active, and how are they organizing the situation?
- What is sacred, threatened, defended, desired, or grieved?
- What is the system unable or unwilling to feel, say, remember, or know?
- How are task, role, authority, and boundary being experienced in feeling rather than only described in words?
- What might recovery of soul look like here, even in a modest and time-limited form?

APPENDIX C. IMPLEMENTING THE RIGHT RESOURCE MODEL: TASK, AUTHORITY, AND COLLABORATION

The Right Resource Model is a way to organize spiritual care capability, not merely a description of chaplaincy identity. It asks who needs what, from whom, at what depth, toward what end, and under whose authority. That last question governs implementation.

An individual chaplain can use the model as a discipline of assessment, restraint, referral, documentation, and consultation. A chaplain can notice a mismatch between need and resource, name a gap, gather cases, and seek authorization for change. A chaplain acting alone cannot redesign a department, reassign work across disciplines, alter credentials or scope, redirect institutional resources, or establish a new delivery system. Right Resource realignment requires formal authority, an institutional sponsor, operational collaboration, and the participation of those whose work will change.

Read Implementation Through TRAB-S

Task

What institutional problem is the realignment meant to address? Is the primary task better patient care, reliable religious accommodation, high-acuity clinical capability, staff support, resource stewardship, or some defined combination? A project that cannot state its primary task will be captured by status anxiety, cost cutting, coverage pressure, or professional self-protection.

Role

Who will sponsor, convene, assess, decide, design, train, supervise, implement, and evaluate? Distinguish the role of executive leadership, spiritual care leadership, clinical chaplains, other chaplains, volunteers, community clergy, nursing, medicine, social work, behavioral health, ethics, palliative care, human resources, and operations as the setting requires. Collaboration becomes confusion when roles remain implicit.

Authority

Who has the right to authorize the work, assign resources, approve policies, define scope, and hold participants accountable? Formal authority must be explicit and accompanied by access, time, information, budget, data, and supervisory support. Personal authority permits participants to contribute judgment and expertise; it does not substitute for delegated institutional authority.

Boundary

Define the population, unit, service line, time period, budget, data set, confidentiality rules, referral criteria, credential limits, ritual authority, and decision rights included in the work. A bounded pilot is usually more learnable than an institution-wide announcement. Hand-offs between volunteers, chaplains, clinical chaplains, community clergy, and interdisciplinary partners require particular attention.

Soul

Realignment touches identity, status, livelihood, vocation, belonging, and fear of replacement. It may mobilize RAGE when authority feels blocked, FEAR about job security, PANIC/GRIEF over a familiar role, CARE for patients and colleagues, PLAY in designing something new, and SEEKING toward greater capability. Treating these responses as mere resistance will reproduce the very system dynamics the model is meant to clarify.

A Collaborative Implementation Sequence

1. Secure authorization and sponsorship

Identify the leader or authorized body that can commission the work, set its limits, supply resources, and act on findings. Clarify what the working group may recommend and what it may decide.

2. Define the primary task and boundaries

Write a short task statement. Name the population, setting, time frame, exclusions, and desired capability. Distinguish improvement of care from defense of a department or profession.

3. Convene the right working group

Include the people who hold relevant authority, operational knowledge, clinical competence, and lived experience. In healthcare this will commonly include spiritual care, executive or operational leadership, nursing or medicine, social work or behavioral health, ethics or palliative care, and volunteer or community-faith representation where appropriate.

4. Map actual needs and current pathways

Use referrals, chart review, cases, interviews, and service data to identify what actually arises. Include religious accommodation, tradition-specific rites, ordinary supportive care, spiritual distress, family and team dynamics, moral distress, trauma, grief, staff needs, and institutional anxiety. Do not begin with services the current staff prefers to provide.

5. Define acuity, competence, role, and authority

Describe which needs may be met by self and family resources, trained volunteers, community clergy or faith representatives, professional chaplains, psychodynamically trained clinical chaplains, and interdisciplinary partners. State the competence and authority required at each level and the limits of every role.

6. Design referral and escalation pathways

Teach referrers to name what they observe rather than request a generic chaplain. Specify how urgent needs are triaged, how high-acuity cases are escalated, how tradition-specific care is obtained, how handoffs occur, and who retains responsibility for follow-up.

7. Pilot within a defined boundary

Test the model in one unit, population, shift, or service line for a stated period. Supply training, supervision, communication, documentation standards, and a way to identify unintended effects.

8. Review cases, data, and consequences

Ask whether the right resource was used, whether acuity was recognized, whether anyone overfunctioned or underfunctioned, whether the patient's symbolic world was respected, and whether continuity improved. Review the effect on workload, access, team understanding, safety, and staff experience.

9. Translate value without reducing the work

Report what leaders need to know: patient and family experience, religious accommodation, care coordination, staff support, moral distress, end-of-life quality, risk, access, and capability. Use numbers where they clarify and cases where they reveal. Translation is necessary; reduction is not.

10. Establish governance, formation, and review

Decide who owns the model, who trains and supervises each resource, how competence is demonstrated, how concerns are escalated, and when the system will be reviewed. Annual review is a minimum; major changes in population, staffing, mission, law, or institutional stress require earlier reconsideration.

What Success Looks Like

Success is not that every stakeholder likes every distinction. It is that the institution can name its spiritual care task, match need and acuity with appropriate competence and authority, protect specialized capacity, provide reliable referral and follow-up, and learn from cases. A sound realignment raises the bar for chaplains by making capability visible. That visibility can strengthen rather than weaken job security: institutions are more likely to value work they can understand, deploy appropriately, and hold accountable.

Practice Implications

> The Right Resource Model becomes institutional practice only when task, role, authority, boundary, and soul are addressed together. Individual chaplains can assess, refer, document, consult, and name gaps. Organizational realignment requires an authorized sponsor, a collaborative working group, a bounded pilot, case-and-data review, and continuing governance. The aim is capability: the right care from the right resource, under the right authority, at the right depth.

APPENDIX D. A MINIMAL READING PATH

This is a path, not a bibliography. It names the smallest sequence I can presently recommend for readers who want to understand the intellectual and clinical world behind this book. One can start anywhere, but it may be helpful to read more or less in order: a first pass for orientation, then a return to the longer works through cases, supervision, and actual questions from practice.

1. The current field statement

HealthCare Chaplaincy Network and Spiritual Care Association, *Psychodynamic Chaplaincy: Psychological and Spiritual Integration in Healthcare*. Read the paper in full. Use it as the concise public statement of the field position from which this book proceeds; then notice where the present manuscript makes the argument more direct, more ecological, and more demanding.

2. The clinical pastoral origin

Anton T. Boisen, *Out of the Depths*. Long out of print but hopefully soon to be republished by Verbum Icon, it should be read as a clinical narrative, not as a founder's relic. Attend to crisis as possible reorganization, to the living human document, and to Boisen's insistence that human lives can become sources of disciplined inquiry. *The Exploration of the Inner World*—the book that established Boisen as the founder of the clinical pastoral movement and charted the course for clinical chaplaincy—is also foundational and, hopefully, soon to be republished. Meanwhile, the classic Boisen reader *Vision from a Little Known Country*, edited by Glenn Asquith and including short works by and about Boisen, will be back in print from Verbum Icon in 2026.

For a concise bridge from Boisen's founding vision to clinical method, read Robert Charles Powell's "'Cooperative Inquiry' in Pastoral Care," collected in his *Anton T. Boisen (1876–1965): Cooperative Inquiry amid the Complex Entanglements of Actual Life*.

3. Assessment, diagnosis, and clinical formulation

Begin with Lynda Juall Carpenito, *Handbook of Nursing Diagnosis*, 14th ed., especially the sections "Spiritual Distress," "Risk for Spiritual Distress," "Impaired Religiosity," and "Risk for Impaired Religiosity," 622–632. Use them for observable characteristics, contributing factors, goals, and interdisciplinary language: a disciplined initial assessment resource, not the endpoint of clinical chaplaincy diagnosis. Then read Paul W. Pruyser, *The Minister as Diagnostician*, as the classic historical statement. His named pastoral diagnoses are too narrow for the ecology developed in this book, but his insistence that ministry requires disciplined diagnostic perception remains foundational. Read both alongside Chapter 9, which moves from screening and inherited categories toward provisional formulation of meaning, affect, relationship, system, and resource fit.

4. Relational use of self

Pamela Cooper-White, *Shared Wisdom: Use of the Self in Pastoral Care and Counseling*, revised and expanded twentieth-anniversary edition.

Read the Introduction and chapters 2, 3, 4, and 6: countertransference and intersubjectivity; pastoral assessment and theological/spiritual reflection; pastoral and spiritual care; and empathy, boundaries, and the special carer. Cooper-White is the preeminent figure in contemporary psychodynamically informed chaplaincy, and much can be gained from her other works, especially *Many Voices: Pastoral Psychotherapy in Relational and Theological Perspective* and *Braided Selves*.

5. The primacy of affect

Mark Solms, *The Hidden Spring*, is the single best source for understanding mind/soul: how feeling defines consciousness and how memory works predictively, both consciously and unconsciously. Solms, a psychoanalyst and neuroscientist who named the emerging field of neuropsychoanalysis, collaborated with the late Jaak Panksepp. Panksepp's *The Archaeology of Mind*, co-written with Lucy Biven, is the key in-depth text for understanding the primary emotional systems. Read the Preface and chapters 1–2, then the opening and concluding sections of chapters 3–10 on SEEKING, RAGE, FEAR, learning and memory, LUST, CARE, PANIC/GRIEF, and PLAY. Return to the full chapters as clinical questions require. Renato Rosaldo's "Grief and the Headhunter's Rage," which opens *Culture and Truth*, powerfully demonstrates the universality of the emotions and the specificity of their expression in different cultures, settings, and circumstances.

6. Religion, symbol, culture, and lived worlds

Clifford Geertz's two indispensable chapters, "Thick Description: Toward an Interpretive Theory of Culture" and "Religion as a Cultural System," are both in *The Interpretation of Cultures*. Carol Delaney's one-of-a-kind anthropology text, *Investigating Culture*, is a treasure trove from cover to cover and includes Jill Dubisch's "You Are What You Eat: Religious Aspects of the Health Food Movement." Read them together: Geertz for definition and method, Delaney for the disciplined work of orientation and disorientation, and Dubisch as a test of whether the reader can recognize religious function outside conventional religious institutions.

7. Cues, clues, and abductive inquiry

Thomas A. Sebeok and Jean Umiker-Sebeok, *You Know My Method: A Juxtaposition of Charles S. Peirce and Sherlock Holmes*. Read the entire short work. Its point for chaplaincy is the disciplined movement from signs to a plausible, testable, and revisable hypothesis. It is a masterpiece in grasping cues and clues.

8. Ecology, context, and the pattern which connects

Nora Bateson, director, *An Ecology of Mind: A Daughter's Portrait of Gregory Bateson* (2010). Watch the film in full. Do not treat it as a substitute for Gregory Bateson or as assigned relief from reading. Let its images, voices, stories, and relationships provide an experiential orientation to context, feedback, difference, learning, and the pattern which connects. Then read *Mind and Nature: A Necessary Unity* as Bateson's mature systematic statement. For shorter points of entry, dip into *Steps to an Ecology of Mind* and *A Sacred Unity: Further Steps to an Ecology of Mind*, especially "A Social Scientist Views the Emotions," "The Moral and Aesthetic Structure of Human Adaptation," "Symptoms, Syndromes, and Systems," and "Seek the Sacred."

9. Human systems from BART to TRAB-S

Zachary Gabriel Green and René J. Molenkamp, "The BART System of Group and Organizational Analysis," https://digital.sandiego.edu/cgi/viewcontent.cgi?article=1084&context=soles-faculty, followed by David Roth, "Consciousness, Soul, and the Architecture of Human Systems: BART Revisited," Clinical Chaplaincy Papers, no. 1 (2025), https://www.clinicalchaplaincy.org/resources. Read both essays in full and in that order. Ask what TRAB-S retains, what it reorders, and what changes when Soul and affect are made explicit.

This learning path is deliberately incomplete. The longer source list that follows identifies further work for citation and study. The minimal path succeeds in practice only if it changes what the reader notices in the next clinical chaplaincy case.

SELECTED BIBLIOGRAPHY

Asquith, Glenn H., Jr., ed. *Vision from a Little Known Country: A Boisen Reader*. Decatur, GA: Journal of Pastoral Care Publications, 1992.

Bateson, Gregory. *Mind and Nature: A Necessary Unity*. New York: E. P. Dutton, 1979.

Bateson, Gregory. *A Sacred Unity: Further Steps to an Ecology of Mind*. Edited by Rodney E. Donaldson. New York: Cornelia & Michael Bessie Books, 1991.

Bateson, Gregory. *Steps to an Ecology of Mind: Collected Essays in Anthropology, Psychiatry, Evolution, and Epistemology*. San Francisco: Chandler Publishing Company, 1972.

Bateson, Nora, dir. *An Ecology of Mind: A Daughter's Portrait of Gregory Bateson*. Bullfrog Films, 2010. Documentary film.

Bion, W. R. *Experiences in Groups and Other Papers*. London: Tavistock Publications, 1961.

Boisen, Anton T. *The Exploration of the Inner World: A Study of Mental Disorder and Religious Experience*. Chicago: Willett, Clark & Co., 1936.

Boisen, Anton T. *Out of the Depths: An Autobiographical Study of Mental Disorder and Religious Experience*. New York: Harper & Brothers, 1960.

Boisen, Anton T. *Religion in Crisis and Custom: A Sociological and Psychological Study*. New York: Harper & Brothers, 1955.

Buirski, Peter, Pamela Haglund, and Emily Markley. *Making Sense Together: The Intersubjective Approach to Psychotherapy*. 2nd ed. Lanham, MD: Rowman & Littlefield, 2020.

Burton, Tara Isabella. "CrossFit Is My Church: How Fitness Classes Provide the Meaning That Religion Once Did." *Vox*, September 10, 2018. https://www.vox.com/the-goods/2018/9/10/17801164/crossfit-soulcycle-religion-church-millennials-casper-ter-kuile.

Carpenito, Lynda Juall. *Handbook of Nursing Diagnosis*. 14th ed. Philadelphia: Lippincott Williams & Wilkins, 2012.

Cooper-White, Pamela. *Braided Selves: Collected Essays on Multiplicity, God, and Persons*. Eugene, OR: Cascade Books, 2011.

Cooper-White, Pamela. *Many Voices: Pastoral Psychotherapy in Relational and Theological Perspective*. Minneapolis: Fortress Press, 2007.

Cooper-White, Pamela. *Shared Wisdom: Use of the Self in Pastoral Care and Counseling*. Revised and expanded 20th anniversary ed. Minneapolis: Fortress Press, 2024.

Delaney, Carol, with Deborah Kaspin. *Investigating Culture: An Experiential Introduction to Anthropology*. 3rd ed. Hoboken, NJ: Wiley-Blackwell, 2017.

Dubisch, Jill. "You Are What You Eat: Religious Aspects of the Health Food Movement." In *Investigating Culture: An Experiential Introduction to Anthropology*, 3rd ed., by Carol Delaney with Deborah Kaspin, 279–88. Hoboken, NJ: Wiley-Blackwell, 2017.

Freud, Sigmund. Letter to C. G. Jung, December 6, 1906. In *The Freud/Jung Letters: The Correspondence between Sigmund Freud and C. G. Jung*, edited by William McGuire, translated by Ralph Manheim and R. F. C. Hull, 12. Princeton, NJ: Princeton University Press, 1974.

Friston, Karl. "The Free-Energy Principle: A Unified Brain Theory?" *Nature Reviews Neuroscience* 11 (2010): 127–38. https://doi.org/10.1038/nrn2787.

Geertz, Clifford. *The Interpretation of Cultures: Selected Essays*. New York: Basic Books, 1973.

Green, Zachary Gabriel, and René J. Molenkamp. "The BART System of Group and Organizational Analysis: Boundary, Authority, Role and Task." 2005. https://digital.sandiego.edu/soles-faculty/78.

Handzo, George F., Kevin J. Flannelly, Taryn Kudler, Sarah L. Fogg, Stephen R. Harding, Yusuf H. Hasan, A. Meigs Ross, and Bonita E. Taylor. "What Do Chaplains Really Do? II. Interventions in the New York Chaplaincy Study." *Journal of Health Care Chaplaincy* 14, no. 1 (2008): 39–56. https://doi.org/10.1080/08854720802053853.

HealthCare Chaplaincy Network and Spiritual Care Association. *Psychodynamic Chaplaincy: Psychological and Spiritual Integration in Healthcare*. New York, April 2025. https://www.clinicalchaplaincy.org/_files/ugd/613716_6f1ffafd26eb4ffb9891c547cdc94d3c.pdf.

Lawrence, Raymond J. *Nine Clinical Cases: The Soul of Pastoral Care and Counseling*. North Charleston, SC: CreateSpace Independent Publishing Platform, 2015.

Lawrence, Raymond J. *Nine More Clinical Cases: Case Studies in Clinical Pastoral Care, Counseling and Psychotherapy*. CPSP Press, 2020.

Lawrence, Raymond J. *Recovery of Soul: A History and Memoir of the Clinical Pastoral Movement*. CPSP Press, 2017.

Massey, Kevin, Marilyn J. D. Barnes, Dana Villines, Julie D. Goldstein, Anna Lee Hisey Pierson, Cheryl Scherer, Betty Vander Laan, and Wm Thomas Summerfelt. "What Do I Do? Developing a Taxonomy of Chaplaincy Activities and Interventions for Spiritual Care in Intensive Care Unit Palliative Care." *BMC Palliative Care* 14 (2015): 10. https://doi.org/10.1186/s12904-015-0008-0.

McWilliams, Nancy. *Psychoanalytic Diagnosis: Understanding Personality Structure in the Clinical Process*. 2nd ed. New York: Guilford Press, 2011.

McWilliams, Nancy. *Psychoanalytic Psychotherapy: A Practitioner's Guide*. New York: Guilford Press, 2004.

McWilliams, Nancy. *Psychoanalytic Supervision*. New York: Guilford Press, 2021.

Nouwen, Henri J. M. "Anton T. Boisen and Theology through Living Human Documents." *Pastoral Psychology* 19, no. 7 (1968): 49–63. https://doi.org/10.1007/BF01788381.

Panksepp, Jaak. *Affective Neuroscience: The Foundations of Human and Animal Emotions*. New York: Oxford University Press, 1998.

Panksepp, Jaak. "The Basic Emotional Circuits of Mammalian Brains: Do Animals Have Affective Lives?" *Neuroscience & Biobehavioral Reviews* 35, no. 9 (2011): 1791–1804. https://doi.org/10.1016/j.neubiorev.2011.08.003.

Panksepp, Jaak, and Lucy Biven. *The Archaeology of Mind: Neuroevolutionary Origins of Human Emotions*. New York: W. W. Norton, 2012.

Powell, Robert Charles. *Anton T. Boisen (1876–1965): Cooperative Inquiry amid the Complex Entanglements of Actual Life*. 2nd ed. CPSP Press, 2021.

Powell, Robert Charles. *Anton T. Boisen (1876–1965): Studying Empirically 'the Complex Entanglements of Actual Life'*. North Charleston, SC: CreateSpace Independent Publishing Platform, 2015.

Powell, Robert Charles. *Anton Theophilus Boisen (1876–1965), Clinician*, parts I–II. Presentations at the National Clinical Training Seminar—West, Malibu, CA, October 8–9, 2012.

Powell, Robert Charles. *Clinical Pastoral Training, Education, and Transformation: The First Fifty Years of Learning through Supervised Encounter with 'Living Human Documents' (1925–1975) and Some Thoughts about the Second Fifty Years (1975–2025).* CPSP Press, 2021.

Powell, Robert Charles. *When Death Is NOT Theoretical: The Readiness of the Music Group 'Queen' for Living with Freddie Mercury's Dying*. 2nd rev. and expanded ed. North Charleston, SC: CreateSpace Independent Publishing Platform, 2018.

Pruyser, Paul W. *The Minister as Diagnostician: Personal Problems in Pastoral Perspective.* Philadelphia: Westminster Press, 1976.

Rosaldo, Renato. *Culture and Truth: The Remaking of Social Analysis.* Boston: Beacon Press, 1989.

Roth, David. "Consciousness, Soul, and the Architecture of Human Systems: BART Revisited." Clinical Chaplaincy Papers, no. 1. ClinicalChaplaincy.org, 2025. https://www.clinicalchaplaincy.org/resources.

Sebeok, Thomas A., and Jean Umiker-Sebeok. *'You Know My Method': A Juxtaposition of Charles S. Peirce and Sherlock Holmes*. Bloomington, IN: Gaslight Publications, 1980.

Solms, Mark, and Oliver Turnbull. *The Brain and the Inner World: An Introduction to the Neuroscience of Subjective Experience*. New York: Other Press, 2002.

Solms, Mark. "The Neurobiological Underpinnings of Psychoanalytic Theory and Therapy." *Frontiers in Behavioral Neuroscience* 12 (2018): 294. https://doi.org/10.3389/fnbeh.2018.00294.

Solms, Mark. *The Hidden Spring: A Journey to the Source of Consciousness*. New York: W. W. Norton, 2021.

ACKNOWLEDGMENTS

A book of this sort is necessarily the product of sustained collaboration over many years.

I am indebted in particular to the many chaplains-in-training and supervisors-in-training I have supervised, as well as the graduate students I have taught, whose lives and work have challenged and informed me over the years. It is impossible to name them all.

Of particular note are my current and past colleagues and collaborators in the Nautilus Pacific Chapter of the College of Pastoral Supervision and Psychotherapy (CPSP). Current members Tony Andrews, Ed Luckett, Sergio Manna, Matt Real, and Pam Washburn, together with the late Wade Wroten, have been my closest collaborators and, equally important, my friends. Within CPSP, I must also mention Grace Jainga. I am grateful as well to Binuta Sudhakeran, whose criticism of portions of an earlier version improved this book. Raymond J. Lawrence, CPSP's founder and general secretary emeritus, was my diplomate supervisor and has long supported me and others in the work of psychodynamically informed chaplaincy in the spirit of Anton T. Boisen. Robert Charles Powell, historian of the clinical pastoral movement, has likewise supported this work. I am indebted to them both.

The opportunity to undertake a fellowship under Jennifer Stuart, with supervision by Laurie J. Wilson, at what was then the NYU Psychoanalytic Institute—now the Psychoanalytic Association of New York—brought both me and my work in chaplaincy into a new relationship with the unconscious.

In 2012, Katie Hodge introduced me to the work of Mark Solms and to the emerging field of neuropsychoanalysis. Mark has described the field as carrying forward Freud's original project by making a place for the soul within neuroscience. Learning from and working with him over the years has been a particular privilege, and his imprint is unmistakable in these pages.

In 2013, Charla Hayden and Jack Lampl, leaders in the field of Group Relations, began working with me and some of my colleagues. That collaboration evolved into a consultant team committed to supporting clinical healthcare chaplains, those they care for, and the institutions they serve. The team, now known as the Soul Group, includes Rebecca Ellison, Mojgan Jahan, Jack Lampl, Lenny Levis, Jaime Romo, Tara Victor, and me. This work has become integral to how I practice clinical chaplaincy, how I train others, and what I have written.

The work of Gregory Bateson and that of his daughter, Nora Bateson—who has sat with my trainees in California—have had an enormous impact on this book and on how I approach my work.

Finally, I return to the beginning. John Valentino launched me into the work of chaplaincy many years ago and pointed me toward Boisen, CPSP, and psychodynamic chaplaincy. The late Glenn Asquith, at the reading of my fourth-unit CPE theory paper, was the first person to encourage me to pursue supervisory training. For the opportunity to take up this work, I am grateful to them both.

www.ingramcontent.com/pod-product-compliance
Lightning Source LLC
LaVergne TN
LVHW022224200926
848481LV00006B/2108
* 9 7 9 8 9 9 6 0 2 4 7 2 8 *